A HISTORY *of the* PENNSYLVANIA HOSPITAL

A HISTORY *of the* PENNSYLVANIA HOSPITAL

KRISTEN A. GRAHAM

THE History PRESS

Published by The History Press
Charleston, SC 29403
www.historypress.net

First published 2008

Manufactured in the United States

ISBN 978.1.59629.567.4

Library of Congress Cataloging-in-Publication Data

Graham, Kristen A.
A history of Pennsylvania Hospital / Kristen A. Graham.
p. ; cm.
Includes bibliographical references.
ISBN 978-1-59629-567-4
1. Pennsylvania Hospital (Philadelphia, Pa.)--History. 2. State hospitals--Pennsylvania--History. I. Title.
[DNLM: 1. Pennsylvania Hospital (Philadelphia, Pa.) 2. Hospitals, State--history--Philadelphia. 3. History, Modern 1601---Philadelphia. WX 28 AP4 P3G 2008]
RA982.P52P46 2008
362.1109748'11--dc22
2008033419

"On Visiting Pennsylvania Hospital"
By Francis Scott Key

Whose fair abode is this? Whose happy lot
Has drawn them in these peaceful shades to rest,
And hear the distant hum of busy life?
The city's noise, its clouds of smoke and dust,
Vainly invade these leafy walls that wave
On high around it, sheltering all within,
And wooing the scared bird to stay its flight
And add its note of joy to bless the scene:
The city's toils, and cares, and strifes are, sure,
Alike excluded here—Content here smiles
And reigns, and leads her vot'ries through the maze
Of flower-embroidered walks to bowers of bliss:
O! 'Tis a sight to warm the hearts of him
Who feels for man, and shares the joys he sees.

(Key, the author of the "Star-Spangled Banner," included this poem in a volume of his work published in 1857.)

CONTENTS

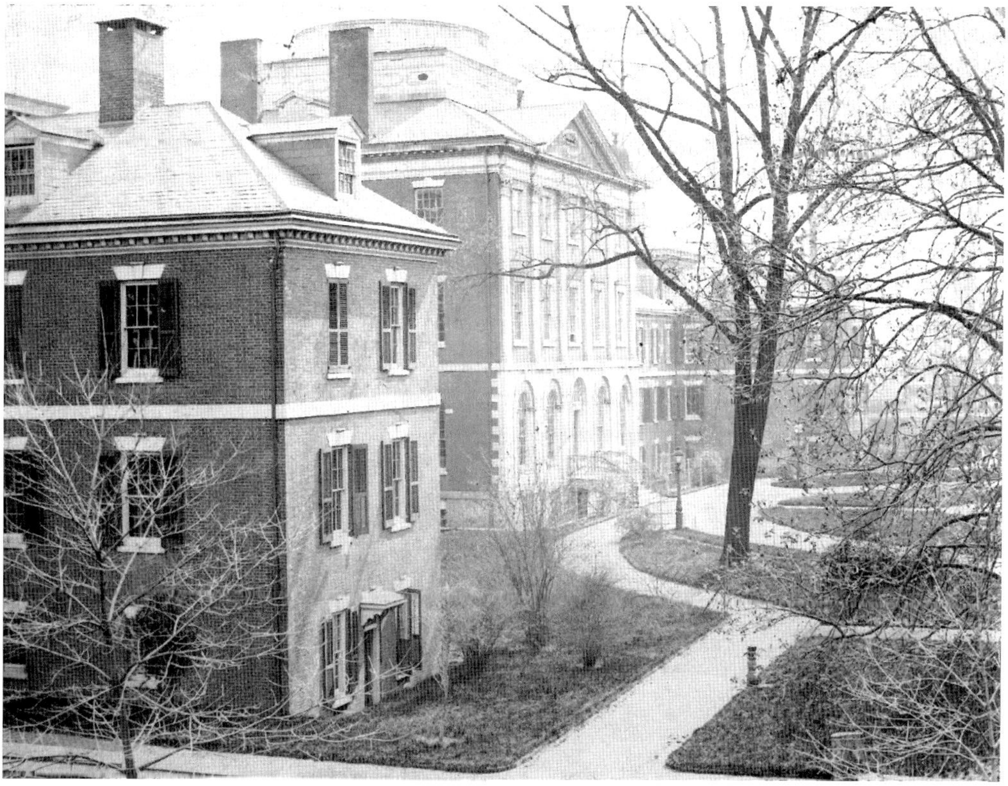

The Pennsylvania Hospital Pine Building. This is the earliest known photograph of the Pine Building, taken by J.C. Browne, April 22, 1861. *Courtesy of the Pennsylvania Hospital, Philadelphia, PAH Image Collection 157.*

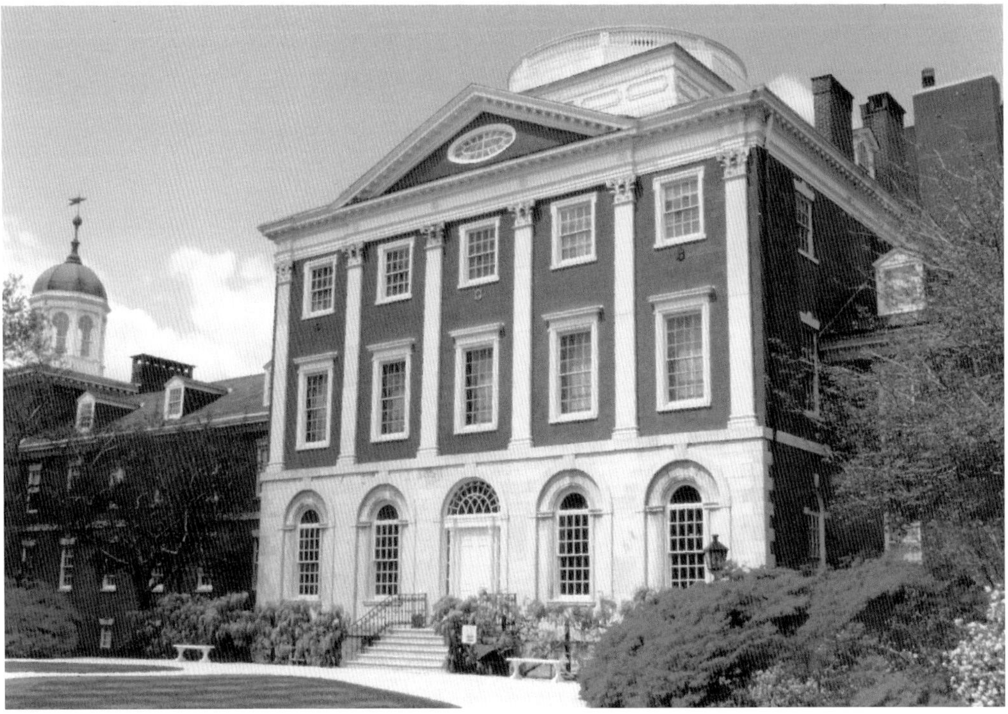

The Pine Building with the wisteria and azaleas in bloom. Tourists make a special trip to see the hospital gardens in full bloom. *Courtesy of the Pennsylvania Hospital, Philadelphia, PAH Image Collection.*

FOREWORD

May 11, 2008, marked the 257th anniversary of the Pennsylvania Hospital. Today, as in 1751, the Pennsylvania Hospital cares for the sick and injured throughout the Philadelphia region. Looking back on such a long history, it is remarkable to consider the number of changes that have taken place—in the city, in healthcare, culturally, socially and economically—yet through all of these changes, the Pennsylvania Hospital has stood the test of time, sometimes coming out on top, other times just getting by, but still standing.

The number of books that have been written about the hospital should number in the hundreds, yet only half a dozen have ever been printed, half of those prior to the twentieth century. Benjamin Franklin, quite appropriately, wrote the first account of the founding in 1754, when he published his *Some Account of the Pennsylvania Hospital*, which was followed up two years later with *A Continuation of Some Account of the Pennsylvania Hospital*. Both were more booklet than book, and they served as development reports to contributors or anyone interested in how the hospital was being run. These accounts, along with all of the early records of the hospital, were taken to an outbuilding during construction in the Historic Library in the mid-nineteenth century; they were rediscovered thirty years later. Upon their discovery, the board of managers resolved to protect them and had them placed in a fireproof vault in the Pine Building.

In 1896, Dr. Thomas Morton, a staff physician and one of those who discovered the historical documents, published what is considered the best account of the hospital. Using these early records, Dr. Morton took great pains to transcribe hundreds of documents in his book. Two other short histories—one celebrating the 150th anniversary of the hospital, and the second, its 200th anniversary—were published by other staff members on their respective anniversaries. The twentieth century saw only two publications regarding the hospital: Dr. Francis Packard published his *Some Account of the Pennsylvania Hospital* in 1936 (a third book by Mrs. Florence Greim continued Dr. Packard's work by bringing it up to 1956), and William Williams published a social history of the hospital in 1976, *The Pennsylvania Hospital, 1751–1801, an internal examination of Anglo-America's first hospital*. Each volume was a unique interpretation of the history of the oldest chartered hospital in the nation.

This newest volume is not meant to reinvent the wheel, but rather to take the best of what has been written, add a little extra and bring the reader to the present. The twentieth century was the scene of many challenges and triumphs for the Pennsylvania Hospital. These stories are told with candor and care. We hope you find this volume accessible, entertaining and educational.

Stacey C. Peeples, Curator-Lead Archivist
Pennsylvania Hospital

AUTHOR'S ACKNOWLEDGEMENTS

This work would not have been possible without the time and effort of many at Pennsylvania Hospital. Stacey Peeples and Mary McCann were my guides from the beginning, and numerous others read early drafts. I'm grateful that their careful work helped tell this important story. I also thank those who shared their own personal recollections about the hospital's past and their observations about its present and future. I appreciate the insights of Dr. Michael Buckley, H. Robert Cathcart, Morris Cheston Jr., Dr. Robert Gill, Kate Kinslow, Dr. Terrence Malloy and Ann Pekarik Stasheff.

For their love and support, thanks are also owed to a legion of family and friends, especially Sam Jacobson, Julia Barth, Amy Graham Barth and Brian Barth. I dedicate this work to Jean Graham and Bill Graham.

INTRODUCTION

Twenty-five years before the United States was formally born at Independence Hall, the nation's first hospital was established by a group of colonists who believed that Philadelphia's citizens deserved a chance to be strong and healthy regardless of their stations in life. It was a radical concept at a time when people who were wealthy and ill were treated at home, while people who were poor and ill languished and often died without care. Even so, Pennsylvania Hospital's founding fathers began with what they thought was a modest enough idea—a small, provincial institution that considered patients on a case-by-case basis.

In the more than 250 years since Dr. Thomas Bond and Benjamin Franklin established the hospital, one constant has been a culture of firsts. In addition to being America's first hospital, Pennsylvania Hospital was also the first place in the country to treat psychological and emotional disorders as curable conditions. It gave America its first apothecary, its first medical resident, its first medical library and its first surgical amphitheatre. In recent years, it has given the world some of the first orthopedic surgery to use a gender-specific artificial knee. Each year, nearly 25,000 patients are admitted into its 515 beds, with an additional 200,000 outpatient visits. And nearly 5,000 babies are born at Eighth and Spruce, the most in the city. Once a modest charity, it has made the transition to a twenty-first-century hospital, a sophisticated, cutting-edge center of innovation and care.

Pennsylvania Hospital has weathered centuries worth of pressures and challenges. It has withstood social and economic transformations, a revolution and both civil and world wars. It has expanded and contracted, opened and closed branches and buildings and started and ended programs as patient, community and regional needs dictated. Its facilities are modern, yet it maintains its Historic Surgical Amphitheatre as a reminder of how far medical practice has come. "It's not just the bricks and mortar," says Kathleen Kinslow, the hospital's executive director. "History is part of what makes up Pennsylvania Hospital, part of everything we do."

THE EARLY HOSPITAL, 1751–1800

ROOTS OF THE NATION'S FIRST HOSPITAL

Philadelphia in 1750 was a boomtown: the largest city in the thirteen colonies, with a population of fifteen thousand. It was a rich, growing and important town, a seaport of note with many "firsts," as well as scientific and cultural institutions. The city was known for its Library Company of Philadelphia (1731), the College of Philadelphia (1749, now the University of Pennsylvania) and the American Philosophical Society (1743).[1] By the eve of the American Revolution, William Penn's "green countrie towne" had become the largest English-speaking city in the British Empire, second only to London. The city boasted a bustling port, and it gained a reputation among foreign visitors as an up-and-coming place. With growth, however, came social ills, including disease and the lack of resources for the "sick poor," affecting needy Philadelphians, but also those passing through the city. Wealthy and middle-class citizens were treated at home—operations were typically performed on kitchen tables—but no such care was available for the neediest class, many of whom suffered and died without aid.[2] Poorhouses, which functioned somewhat like today's homeless shelters, were the only quasi-medical facilities available to the masses,[3] and the closest hospitals were in Mexico City (established in 1524) and Quebec (established in 1639).

Keen observers noted the problem. In 1709, a group of Quakers discussed establishing a hospital, but the idea went nowhere.[4] In 1731, Benjamin Franklin's *Pennsylvania Gazette* implored readers to exercise "a tender regard for the afflicted [with disease]."[5] But no specific mention of the need for a hospital was made, despite the fact that a surge of such institutions was afoot in England. Twenty years later, however, a similar appeal was made, this time with a note that the notion of "an institution of the same kind [hospital] has met with such encouragement in Pennsylvania…that there is reason to expect it may be carried into execution the ensueing year."[6]

DR. BOND STIRS UP SUPPORT

The seed of the idea for America's first hospital came from Dr. Thomas Bond, a prominent Philadelphian whose civic ideals drove him to help establish the College of Philadelphia and the American Philosophical Society. He drew inspiration from a new kind of hospital cropping up in Great Britain—hospitals that were established and maintained by voluntary contributions, existing for the purpose of providing care for the poor.[7] News accounts detailing the workings of such "voluntary" hospitals had been readily available to colonists since the 1730s. And among many Quaker Philadelphians, there was both a drive for better medical knowledge and a desire to better the situations of the sick poor, though less out of a spirit of pure generosity than from a desire to give deserving paupers the tools—namely, good health—to pull themselves out of poverty.[8] Philadelphia did have an almshouse, established in 1731, but it was little more than a warehouse for the aged and infirm poor.[9]

Dr. Bond, who became impressed with European hospitals during his training there, had served as Philadelphia's port inspector in the 1740s and was convinced that the city needed its own voluntary hospital. The port inspector job—crucial in a seaport such as Philadelphia—made him aware of the increasing prevalence of diseases brought in by the ships that came to the city, ailments such as cholera, typhus, smallpox and bubonic plague. In 1750, Dr. Bond began to secure funding for a hospital, which he believed would help in the treatment and quarantine of sufferers of these diseases. Such an institution could also serve the mentally ill, many who in those days simply wandered the streets.

At first, Dr. Bond struggled to muster support for his plan; potential donors often asked him about the position of one of the most important men in the colonies, Dr. Bond's friend Benjamin Franklin. Dr. Bond initially told them he had not approached Franklin, feeling that it was somewhat out of his range of interest. But it quickly became apparent that there might be no hospital without Franklin's support, so Dr. Bond approached his friend. Franklin asked for details of the plan and, in short order, became both a subscriber and the person who would help sway opinion among legislators and the public.[10] In fact, Franklin's autobiography affirms both the genesis of the idea of Pennsylvania Hospital and his support for it: "Dr. Thomas Bond a particular friend of mine, conceived the idea of establishing a hospital in Philadelphia for the reception and cure of poor sick persons…a very beneficent design, which has been ascribed to me but was originally his."

POLITICS AND ORGANIZING: THE HOSPITAL'S FIRST DAYS

In January 1751, the Provincial Assembly of Pennsylvania received a petition from "sundry inhabitants of the said Province" seeking authority to establish a hospital for the poor, sick, injured and these "distemper'd in Mind and deprived of their rational Faculties," whose numbers "hath greatly increased in this Province," in addition to which "many languish out their Lives, tortur'd perhaps with the Stone, devour'd by the Cancer, deprived of Sight by Cataracts, or gradually decaying by loathsome Distempers."[11]

The petition was written in Franklin's handwriting, but his signature was not among those listed. Still, his work behind the scenes was key to the political maneuvering necessary to get the hospital off the ground. Within a week, a bill that would establish just such a hospital was introduced to the assembly. Franklin engineered a plan that was difficult to resist, even for rural legislators who were reluctant to approve a city hospital: contributors were to meet, choose managers and a treasurer and to raise £2,000, a sum that some thought was out of reach. Once the sum was raised, Franklin suggested, the assembly would match the voluntary subscriptions. This was almost certainly the first time that a matching-funds drive was launched in America.

Franklin and his cohorts exceeded their goal, gathering £2,751, the assembly approved the measure and on May 11, 1751, Pennsylvania Hospital was established with the signature of Lieutenant Governor James Hamilton.[12] Franklin later wrote: "I do not remember any of my political manoeuvres, the success of which gave me at the time more pleasure."

The first formal assembly of the contributors to the hospital was held two months later on July 1, 1751. Meeting in the city's statehouse, later to gain fame as Independence Hall,

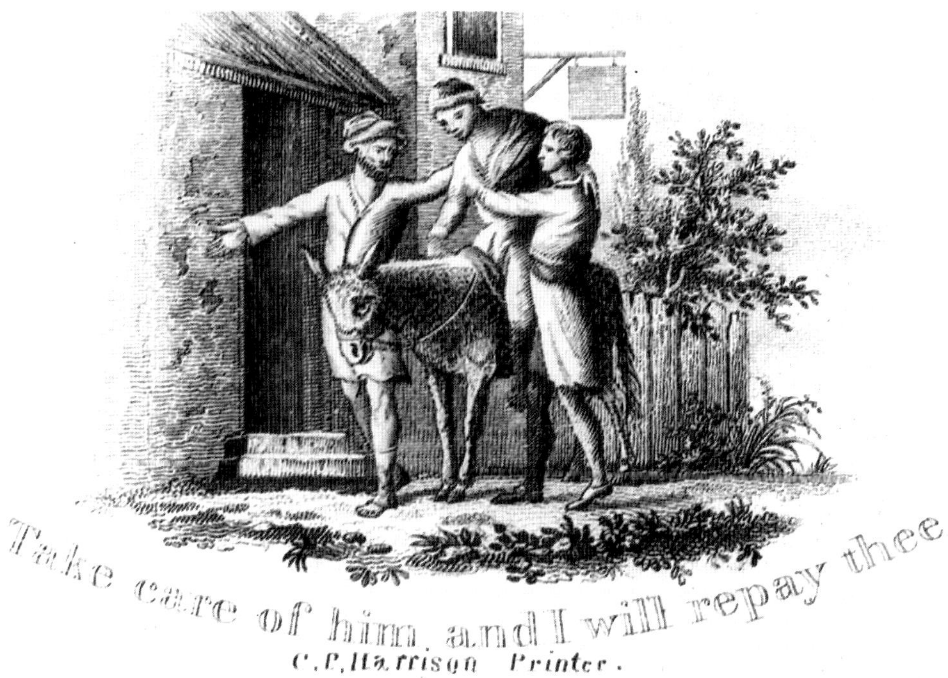

The board of managers elected Dr. Thomas Bond and Benjamin Franklin to decide on a logo for the hospital. They chose the story of the Good Samaritan. Here, the Samaritan is seen taking an injured man to an inn for aid, with the saying, "Take care of him and I will repay thee." This image can still be found throughout the hospital campus. *Courtesy of the Pennsylvania Hospital, Philadelphia, PAH Image Collection 1609.*

the group chose twelve managers and a treasurer, noting that the officeholders would remain until the "first second day in the Month called May," a tradition that still holds. The managers were among the most prominent men in Philadelphia—apart from Bond and Franklin, they were wealthy merchants like Samuel Hazard and Israel Pemberton, or civically active clergymen such as Richard Peters. The managers chose Joshua Crosby from among their ranks to serve as president, and picked Benjamin Franklin as clerk. Later, they would adopt a rule that any manager who was late to a meeting would pay a fine of one shilling; an absence would cost him two shillings. Dr. Bond, the only physician to serve on the board (he resigned when he was appointed to the staff of the hospital), and Franklin were given the task of preparing a seal for the new hospital, and they chose one depicting the biblical story of the Good Samaritan helping a sick man to an inn. "Take care of him, and I will repay thee," it read. Bond, his brother Phineas and Lloyd Zachary were soon appointed to the first medical staff.

In the early days of the hospital, the managers drew up rules for its medical staff, stating that six "practitioners of Physick & Surgery" would be chosen each May. Those physicians were asked to "keep a fair account [in a book provided for that purpose] of the several Patients under their Care, of the Disorders they labour under & shall enter in the said book the Recipes or Prescriptions they make for each of them." Physicians had to be at least twenty-seven years old, to have served a regular apprenticeship in the city or suburbs, to have studied for seven or more years and to submit to an examination by hospital doctors in the presence of the managers. They had to reside in the city for at least three years.[13]

RUNNING A HOSPITAL

The first order of business was to secure a suitable place to run a hospital. The managers chose a large house on the south side of High Street, now Market, below Seventh. They rented the house, with its gardens, stable and roomy, airy interiors, from the estate of the late Judge John Kinsey. The cost was forty pounds for eighteen months

On February 6, 1752, an item ran in the *Pennsylvania Gazette* announcing that the Pennsylvania Hospital was ready to accept patients and that "Israel Pemberton and Dr. Thomas Bond have secured a suitable matron to take care of the house and of the Sick that shall be placed there." Quaker widow Elizabeth Gardner was hired at twenty shillings a year. Four days later, the managers met to discuss the first applicants for admittance to the hospital. The mostly Quaker board wanted to know: If the prospective patient was able to work, was he working? Could a hospital stay restore the applicant's health to the point where he could work? The managers wanted to steer away from treating those they considered undeserving. Those who wanted to be patients at Pennsylvania Hospital had to have two tax-paying citizens to sponsor them so that there was a way to provide "burial or travel deposits to indemnify the hospital, either from the expense of burial in case they die, or to defray the expense of carrying them back to their place of abode, that they may not become a charge to the city."

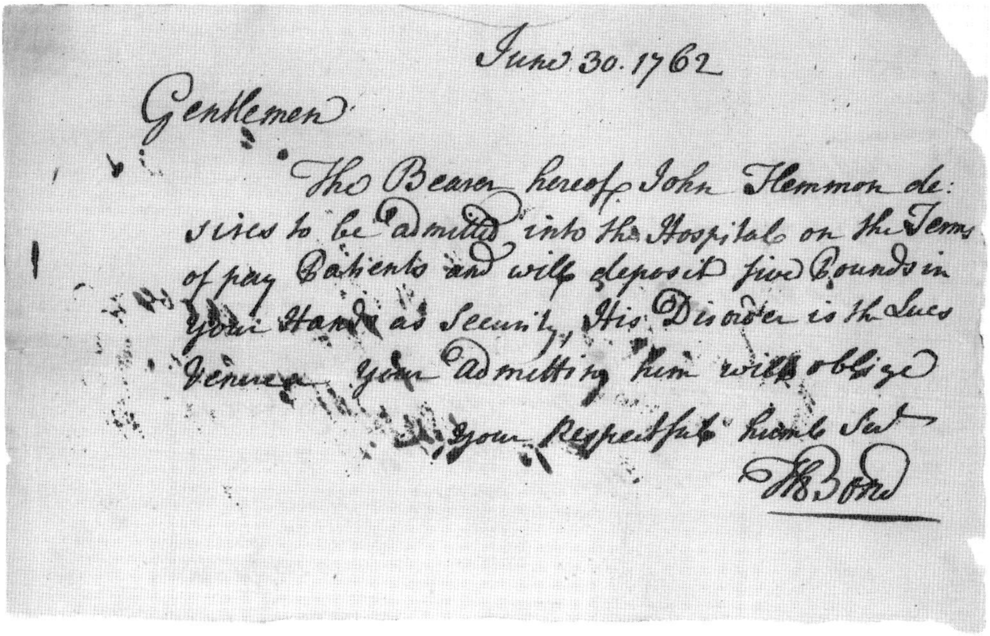

June 30. 1762

Gentlemen

The Bearer hereof John Hemmon desires to be admitted into the Hospital on the Terms of pay Patients and will deposit five Pounds in your Hands as Security, His Disorder is the Lues Venerea your admitting him will oblige

Your Respectfull humble Servt

Th Bond

A patient admission form signed by Dr. Thomas Bond, founder of the Pennsylvania Hospital. *Courtesy of the Pennsylvania Hospital, Philadelphia, Patient Records Collection.*

Funds for patient care often came from the managers themselves, or other philanthropists, but some paying patients (who were asked to pay "such reasonable rates as they can agree for") were accepted if space allowed. (In the late eighteenth century, the managers demanded written testimonial from a "respectable" person attesting to the moral worth of an applicant before he or she was admitted.)

The managers drew up a set of rules for patients in January 1752. They decided to refuse admission to three types of patients—all those judged incurable, except lunatics; all those suffering from smallpox, "itch or other infectious distemper" until proper departments were built; and women with young children, unless the children were taken care of elsewhere. Some of the rules established by the board included: no talking on the ward when physicians were present; no gambling, spitting or swearing; those who were able must help the nurses care for other, sicker patients; and no street clothes (when in bed, patients must wear bedclothes). Patients were also prohibited from leaving the hospital without permission, which must have been a problem, as early records often show the term "eloped" next to patients' names.[14] The managers also asked that when patients were cured, they sign documents testifying to the details of their cases and the benefits they received at the hospital. Those documents could be published or used as the managers saw fit.[15]

Of the initial applicants, two were rejected, and two were admitted to the hospital on February 10, 1752.[16] The first patient was Margaret Sherlock. "Her disorder being a prolepsis uteri," Franklin wrote. Next was Hannah Shines, "a lunatic." Sherlock was discharged a few weeks later, and persuaded the board to hire her as a nurse. The board was open-minded in its admissions, selecting as patients in the first year a black slave and a Native American who was found lying ill near the house of Isaac Norris. Norris was Speaker (1751–66) of the Provincial Assembly of Pennsylvania and for a time served as mayor of Philadelphia. Indeed, the managers were generally intent on treating all patients equally, regardless of class or color. From the minutes of February 20, 1768, the board declared, "That the Pay Patients now in the House and those who are hereafter Admitted be accommodated with no other Provisions for their Diet than the Other Patients, and any Extraordinary necessaries they require, Such as Tea, Loaf Sugar, Coffee, Chocolate, Wine or Spirits, they provide at their own Expense."[17]

The first medicines and medical supplies were contributed by members of the medical staff, but this was only a temporary arrangement.[18] In December 1752, Benjamin Franklin noted, the managers opened a proper apothecary's shop in Pennsylvania Hospital. They appointed Jonathan Roberts apothecary, charged with attending and making up medicines daily, "according to the prescriptions, with an allowance of fifteen pounds per annum for his care and trouble." The medicines in Roberts's shop cost "one hundred twelve pounds, fifteen shillings, and two pence half-penny, sterling," and to pay for these, the managers were instructed to solicit subscriptions from "charitable widows and other good women of the city."[19]

The managers saw this as another stopgap measure, though, and resolved in the future to only spend as much money on medicine as was on hand in the hospital treasury. In 1758, physicians were invited to weigh in on the next year's apothecary, as they now believed a medical student could successfully run the apothecary shop. This meant that the managers no longer had the apothecary's salary to pay. This experiment did not last long, however; by 1767, the managers were advertising for a qualified apothecary. From the hospital's rules and regulations came these duties for the apothecary:

> *He shall reside in the Hospital and perform all the duties appertaining to his department*[;] *He shall keep a meteorological record noting the measurement of the thermometer, barometer, and other meteorological instruments at stated times of each day*[; and] *He shall not absent himself from the Hospital without notifying the Steward, and having his place supplied by one of the Resident Physicians, or such other persons as shall be approved by the Committee.*[20]

While they juggled the job of running a hospital, the managers also sought to find a permanent home for the institution. When the proprietors of Pennsylvania, Thomas and Richard Penn, declined to give the managers land, the board moved to purchase a plot on its own. On September 11, 1754, they bought part of the land now occupied by Pennsylvania Hospital—a parcel running along the north side of Pine Street between Eighth and Ninth Streets. Some objected to the location because it was distant from the center of the city, surrounded by farmland and somewhat difficult to access from the residential and commercial centers of town. Still, the managers considered the ground they chose the best spot for their new hospital, despite its rural setting.

Until the early twentieth century, a large farm bell rang at 6:00 a.m., noon and 6:00 p.m.; it rang not, as tradition later suggested, to announce the distribution of a portion

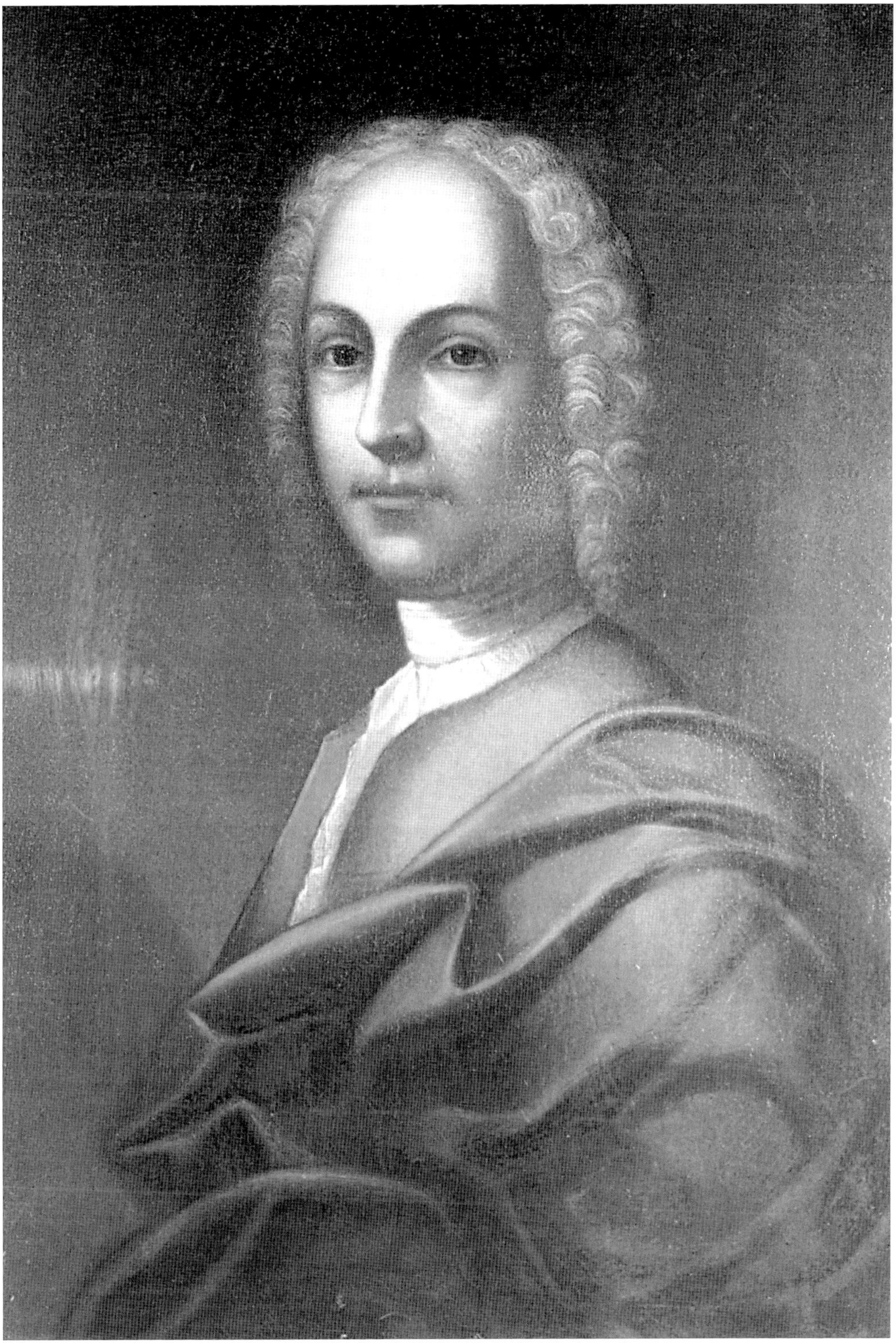

Portrait of Lloyd Zachary, one of the first three physicians at the Pennsylvania Hospital. Along with Dr. Bond, Dr. Zachary and Dr. Phineas Bond (Thomas's brother) worked for no pay for the first three years the hospital was open. *Courtesy of the Pennsylvania Hospital, Philadelphia, PAH Image Collection 1690.*

of rum, but instead to call hospital workers to eat. In keeping with the rural flavor of the place, there were also several hitching posts for horses. They were used until the early twentieth century by Dr. George Harlan, a Pennsylvania Hospital ophthalmologist, who had been a cavalry officer during the Civil War. Dr. Harlan, a serious horseman, used to ride a horse that was reputedly quite spirited to work at the hospital. He died from a fall from this horse in 1909.[21]

A Permanent Home

Later, in 1767, the Penns did present the board an adjacent plot, extending the hospital's grounds to Spruce Street between Eighth and Ninth. But at the time of the purchase, the board named one of its original managers, Samuel Rhoads, later mayor of Philadelphia and at the time an architect with the Carpenter Company, to draw up a plan for the new building. Rhoads envisioned a Georgian structure with three separate wings. (The first part, nearest Eighth Street, was completed in 1755; the West Wing would not be finished until 1797; and the Center Building would be completed in 1804.) On May 28, 1755, the cornerstone was laid with much fanfare—citizens, including the managers, physicians, many contributors of the hospital and many children (the public schools had been dismissed), marched together from the temporary hospital to the site of the new building. The words etched on the cornerstone were Franklin's. He wrote:

In the year of Christ
1755
George the second happily
reigning;
(For he sought the Happiness of
his People)
Philadelphia flourishing,
(For its Inhabitants were
publick-spirited)
This Building,
By the Bounty of the
Government,
And of many private Persons,
Was piously founded,
May the God of Mercies
Bless the Undertaking!

Soon after the cornerstone was laid, Joshua Crosby, the first president of the board of managers, died, and Benjamin Franklin was elected to replace him. Building continued, and on December 17, 1756, all patients were moved from the temporary hospital to

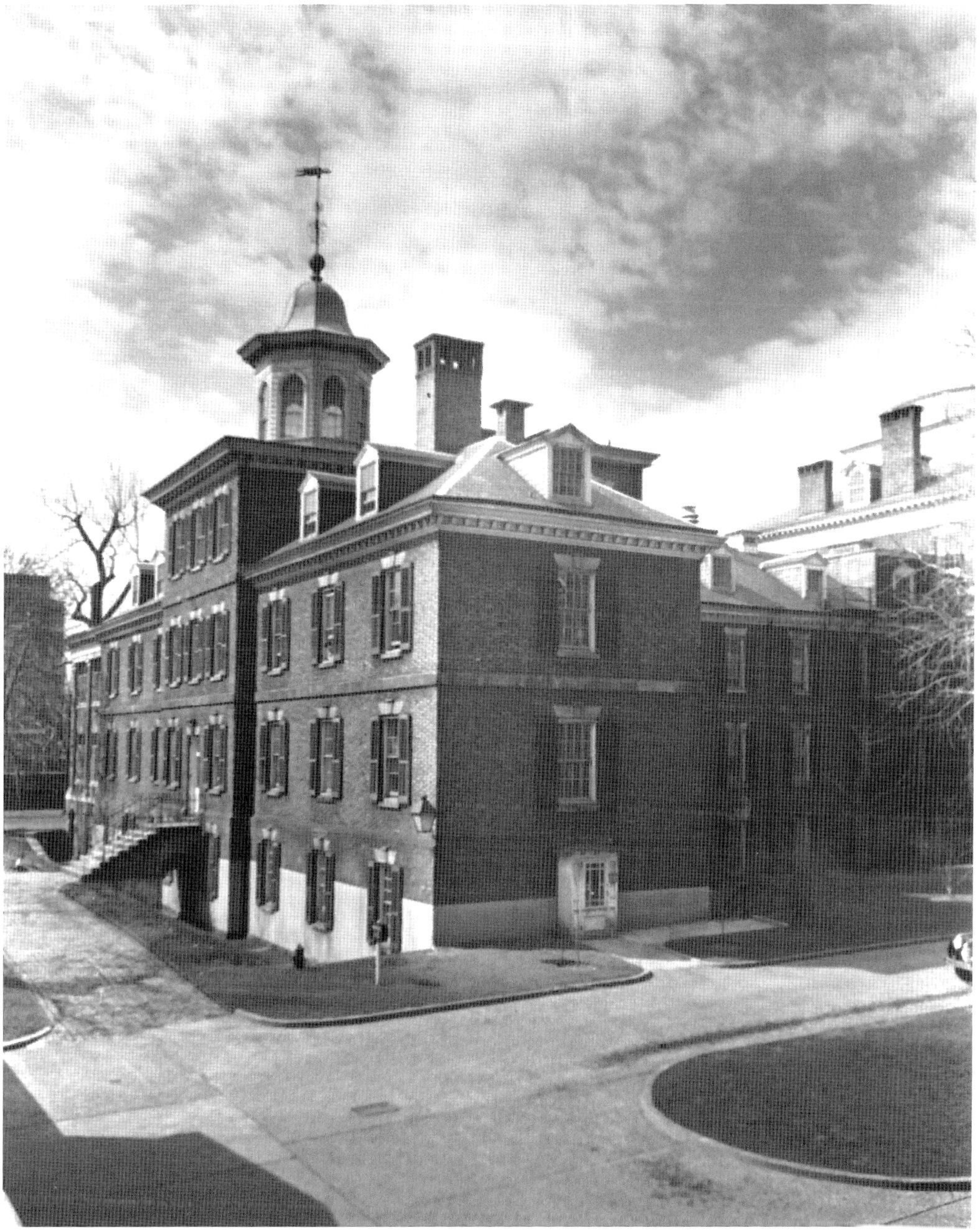

The East Wing Pine Building as it was in the 1950s. To the left is the former main entrance to the hospital. *Courtesy of the Pennsylvania Hospital, Philadelphia, PAH Image Collection.*

the location Pennsylvania Hospital still occupies.[22] Fiscally, the hospital was relatively healthy from its inception through the American Revolution. Despite needing to raise construction funds to pay for the new building, there was generally enough money to treat seventy patients at a time, gratis.

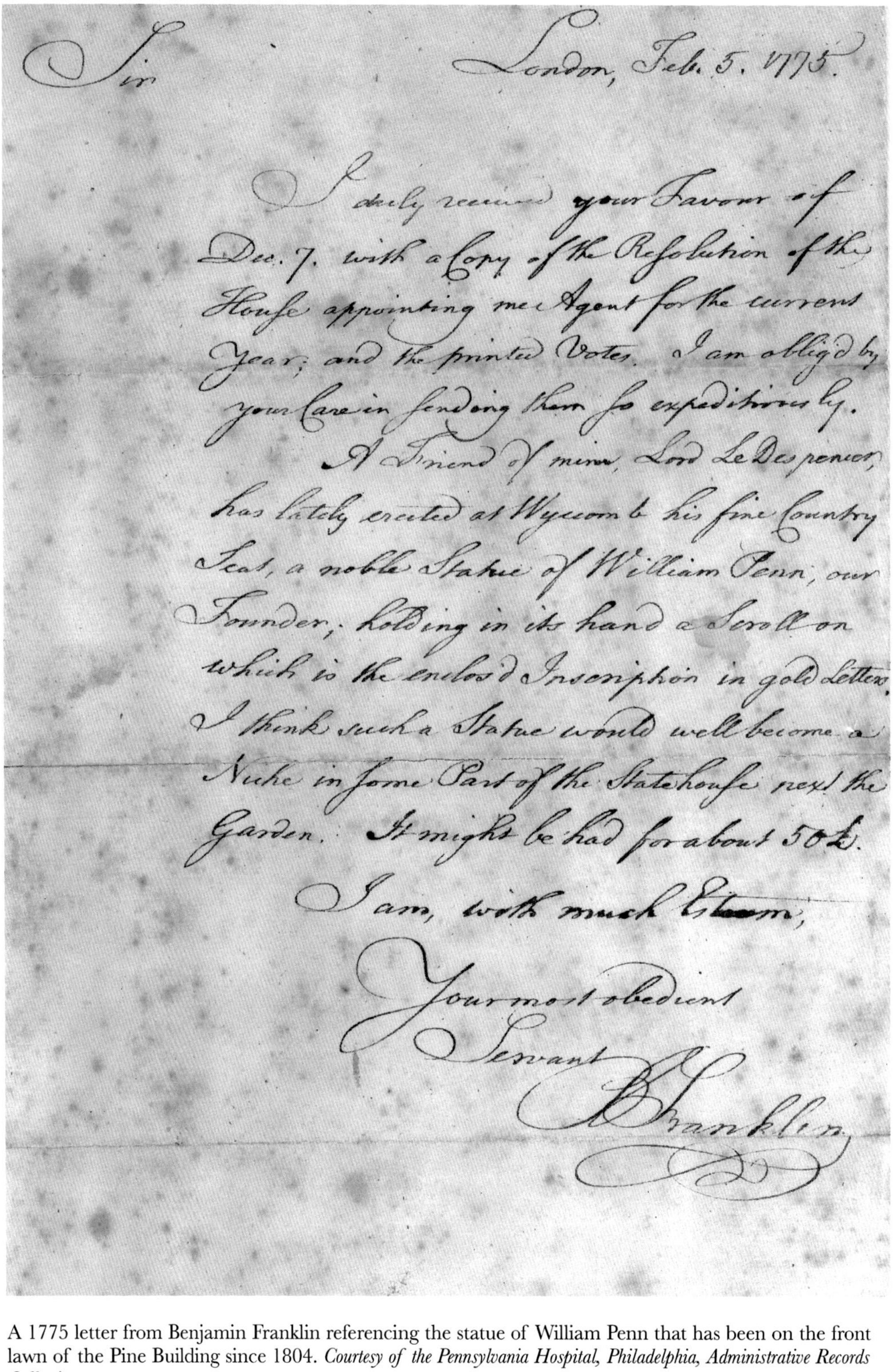

Sir

London, Feb. 5. 1775.

I duly receiv'd your Favour of Dec. 7. with a Copy of the Resolution of the House appointing me Agent for the current Year; and the printed Votes. I am oblig'd by your Care in sending them so expeditiously.

A Friend of mine, Lord Le Despencer, has lately erected at Wycomb his fine Country Seat, a noble Statue of William Penn, our Founder, holding in its hand a Scroll on which is the enclos'd Inscription in gold Letters. I think such a Statue would well become a Niche in some Part of the Statehouse next the Garden. It might be had for about 50£.

I am, with much Esteem,

Your most obedient
Servant
B Franklin

A 1775 letter from Benjamin Franklin referencing the statue of William Penn that has been on the front lawn of the Pine Building since 1804. *Courtesy of the Pennsylvania Hospital, Philadelphia, Administrative Records Collection.*

A boost to the Pennsylvania Hospital treasury came early on, in the form of Franklin's writings. At first, he used his *Pennsylvania Gazette* to broadcast the good works and its need for financial support. But in 1753, the managers directed him to prepare "a full account of the affairs of the Hospital…to be laid before the Assembly." Franklin wrote *Some Account of Pennsylvania Hospital from its First Beginning to the Fifth Month, called May, 1754*—a volume that was not strictly a historical work so much as it was a support-gathering device. *Some Account*, forty pages in all, even included a contribution form to facilitate donations.

The work did have an effect—by August 1754, the board noted that several new subscriptions had been made since its last meeting, and by April of the next year, Pennsylvania Hospital had 186 new subscribers who donated over £2,000 to the capital stock. For the entire year before the publication of *Some Account*, only one new subscriber was reported. Franklin devised other ways of fundraising, too. In 1752, he proposed that boxes be set up for hospital donations, an idea that the board adopted immediately. The charity boxes were placed in the hospital, in homes and in other public places. From 1753 to 1775, they produced more than £900 of revenue.[23]

Increasing operating costs and building expenses still caused a bumpy fiscal road for a time, and in 1761, the assembly granted the hospital £3,000 to replenish its capital stock. This grant inspired new giving among private contributors, and by 1763, the financial ship was righted. Medically speaking, the colonial hospital was coming into its own. Every year, six physicians were selected—men who had to contribute at least £10 to the hospital, spend some time as apprentices in the Philadelphia area, pass an examination and spend seven years or more studying physic (i.e., medicine). Even those with impressive foreign credentials had to live in Philadelphia for three years before they could be considered. Still, in general, the colonial physician was not well educated; by 1775, of the thirty-five hundred practicing physicians in America, four hundred or fewer had attended medical school either in the colonies or abroad. Physicians generally learned by observation and practice.

THE FRENCH AND INDIAN WAR

In 1755, Pennsylvania Hospital received its first war casualties—soldiers who were wounded in the French and Indian War. The hospital received patients involved in battles in western Pennsylvania. "Michael Higgins a Soldier, having his under Jaw shot off in the late Engagem't under General Braddock was admitted an Out-Patient."[24] As was the case in all wars, disease was as problematic to the soldiers as was combat. On December 24, 1758, "Admitted John Brown with an autumnal fever and George Wood with a fever: these two are Captives lately released from Canada."[25]

MEDICAL LECTURES

Medical students were part of the hospital from its earliest days, though formal medical instruction did not begin at Pennsylvania Hospital until 1763. Hospital physicians could and did bring their apprentices to the wards with them. Even apprentices of non-hospital physicians could observe in the wards, provided they paid a fee—six pistoles. In the winter of 1765–66, thirteen students, including Benjamin Rush and William Bartram, son of the famous botanist John Bartram, walked the halls of Pennsylvania Hospital.

The first formal medical lectures were given at the hospital in 1763. A year earlier, Dr. John Fothergill, who would also donate the first book to establish the medical library, sent "some pretty accurate anatomical drawings about half as big as life"[26] to Pennsylvania Hospital with Dr. William Shippen Jr., who was finishing his medical education in Great Britain. Dr. Shippen presented the managers with the drawings and requested the use of the drawings in order to "exhibit a course of lectures on anatomy this winter." The managers agreed, under the conditions that the lectures be held in the hospital and that the fee of one pistole per lecture be charged, with proceeds going to the hospital.

Beginning on May 21, and every two weeks thereafter, Dr. Shippen lectured to "students in physic" and others interested in a "general knowledge of the human body." Dr. Shippen lectured at Pennsylvania Hospital until 1765, when he and Dr. John Morgan founded the new medical school at the College of Philadelphia, the nation's first medical school, later known as the University of Pennsylvania. He moved his lectures there.

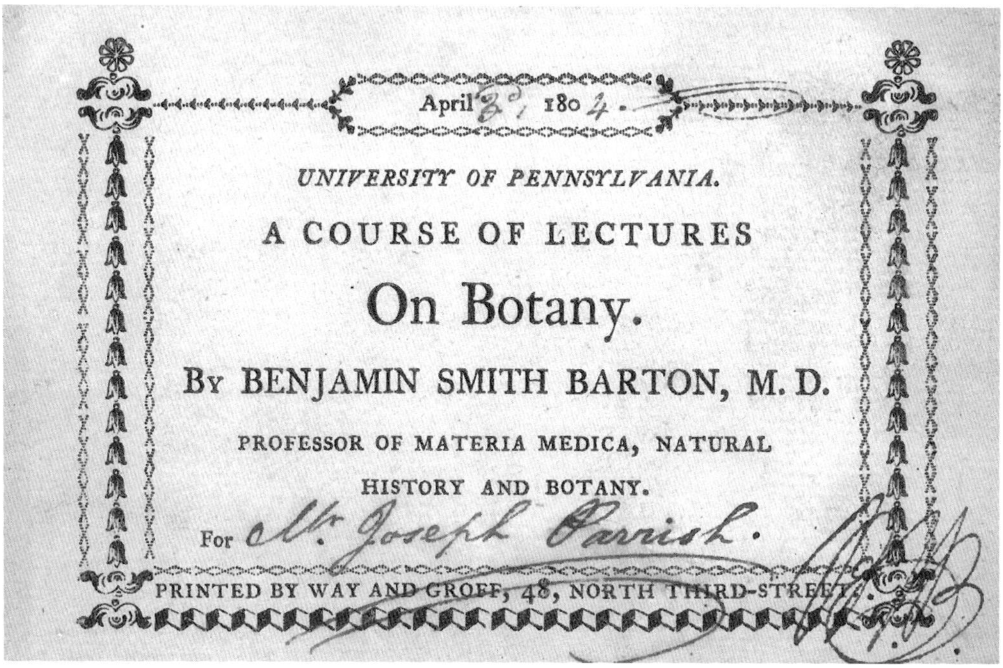

April 30, 1804.

UNIVERSITY OF PENNSYLVANIA.

A COURSE OF LECTURES

On Botany.

By BENJAMIN SMITH BARTON, M. D.

PROFESSOR OF MATERIA MEDICA, NATURAL HISTORY AND BOTANY.

For Mr. Joseph Parrish.

PRINTED BY WAY AND GROFF, 48, NORTH THIRD-STREET.

Medical student Joseph Parrish's admission card to a lecture on botany given by Dr. Benjamin Smith Barton. *Courtesy of the Pennsylvania Hospital, Philadelphia, Administrative Records Collection.*

Once Dr. Shippen—who would return to the hospital, winning appointment to the medical staff in 1778—left, the managers asked Dr. Thomas Bond to begin lectures. His lectures were remarkable because they sparked the staff to allow postmortem dissection, a practice that was largely frowned upon. Conventional wisdom likened dissections to grave robbing and body snatching. But Dr. Bond saw the medical value in the practice, and at his urging, the practice was standardized.[27]

As a physician and scientist, Dr. Bond was remarkable. He was renowned for performing the first lithotomy—removal of a stone from the bladder—in the country, and was also known for a splint for forearm fractures that was used until early in the twentieth century. Dr. Bond was also interested in the weather and presented Pennsylvania Hospital with a meteorological device used to record temperatures. Its product was the first systematic and continuous weather records known to be kept in America. There is some evidence that these records were used in court in cases in which questions about weather conditions arose.[28]

MEDICAL EDUCATION: AMERICA'S FIRST MEDICAL RESIDENT

In the earliest days of the hospital, there was no formal training program for medical students. Doctors would sometimes have the assistance of their own private students, or apothecaries or apprentices, but there were no residencies. That changed in 1773, when Jacob Ehrenzeller Sr., a Philadelphia tavern owner, apprenticed his son, sixteen-year-old Jacob Jr., as Pennsylvania Hospital's first medical resident. Under the terms of his indenture, Ehrenzeller was forbidden to fornicate, buy or sell goods, play cards or run away. It was also stated clearly in the contract that he was to receive special training:

> *That he shall leave at his own or his father's expense to attend the lectures of the Medical Professors out of the Hospital during the last two years of his Apprenticeship; to attend the Surgical Operations and Lectures in the Hospital free of any expense; and that the Apothecary for the time being shall duly instruct him in Physic and Surgery.*

Young Ehrenzeller was, in fact, a first in the colonies—a student who would combine clinical experience (at Pennsylvania Hospital) with studies (at the College of Philadelphia). Ehrenzeller earned a certificate of medical competency from the hospital, but he did not obtain a degree in medicine from the college because classes were suspended in 1777, when the British occupied Philadelphia. No replacement for him was made at the hospital until 1786, when William Gardner was indentured there. This particular practice continued until 1824, when it was decided that residents would need medical degrees.

This tradition continues today, with the names of each resident who has passed through Pennsylvania Hospital's doors—now both men and women—inscribed on plaques on

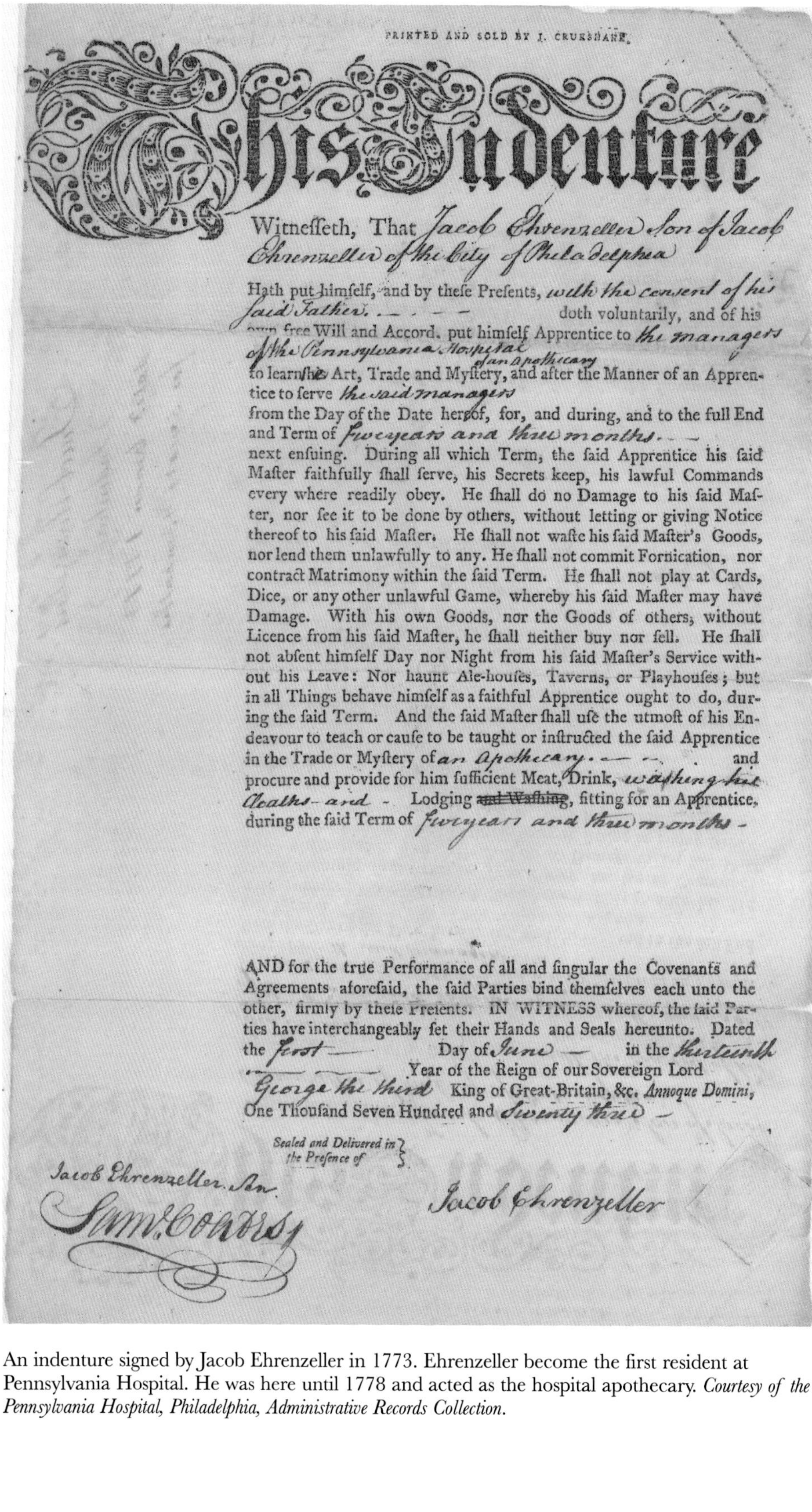
PRINTED AND SOLD BY J. CRUKSHANK.

This Indenture

Witnesseth, That Jacob Ehrenzeller Son of Jacob Ehrenzeller of the City of Philadelphia

Hath put himself, and by these Presents, with the consent of his said Father. — — — doth voluntarily, and of his own free Will and Accord, put himself Apprentice to the managers of the Pennsylvania Hospital to learn the Art, Trade and Mystery, of an Apothecary and after the Manner of an Apprentice to serve the said managers from the Day of the Date hereof, for, and during, and to the full End and Term of five years and three months. — next ensuing. During all which Term, the said Apprentice his said Master faithfully shall serve, his Secrets keep, his lawful Commands every where readily obey. He shall do no Damage to his said Master, nor see it to be done by others, without letting or giving Notice thereof to his said Master. He shall not waste his said Master's Goods, nor lend them unlawfully to any. He shall not commit Fornication, nor contract Matrimony within the said Term. He shall not play at Cards, Dice, or any other unlawful Game, whereby his said Master may have Damage. With his own Goods, nor the Goods of others, without Licence from his said Master, he shall neither buy nor sell. He shall not absent himself Day nor Night from his said Master's Service without his Leave: Nor haunt Ale-houses, Taverns, or Playhouses; but in all Things behave himself as a faithful Apprentice ought to do, during the said Term. And the said Master shall use the utmost of his Endeavour to teach or cause to be taught or instructed the said Apprentice in the Trade or Mystery of an Apothecary. — — and procure and provide for him sufficient Meat, Drink, washing his Cloaths — and — Lodging ~~and Washing~~, fitting for an Apprentice, during the said Term of five years and three months —

AND for the true Performance of all and singular the Covenants and Agreements aforesaid, the said Parties bind themselves each unto the other, firmly by these Presents. IN WITNESS whereof, the said Parties have interchangeably set their Hands and Seals hereunto. Dated the first — Day of June — in the thirteenth — — Year of the Reign of our Sovereign Lord George the third King of Great-Britain, &c. Annoque Domini, One Thousand Seven Hundred and Seventy three —

Sealed and Delivered in the Presence of

Jacob Ehrenzeller. Son

Saml. Coates

Jacob Ehrenzeller

An indenture signed by Jacob Ehrenzeller in 1773. Ehrenzeller become the first resident at Pennsylvania Hospital. He was here until 1778 and acted as the hospital apothecary. *Courtesy of the Pennsylvania Hospital, Philadelphia, Administrative Records Collection.*

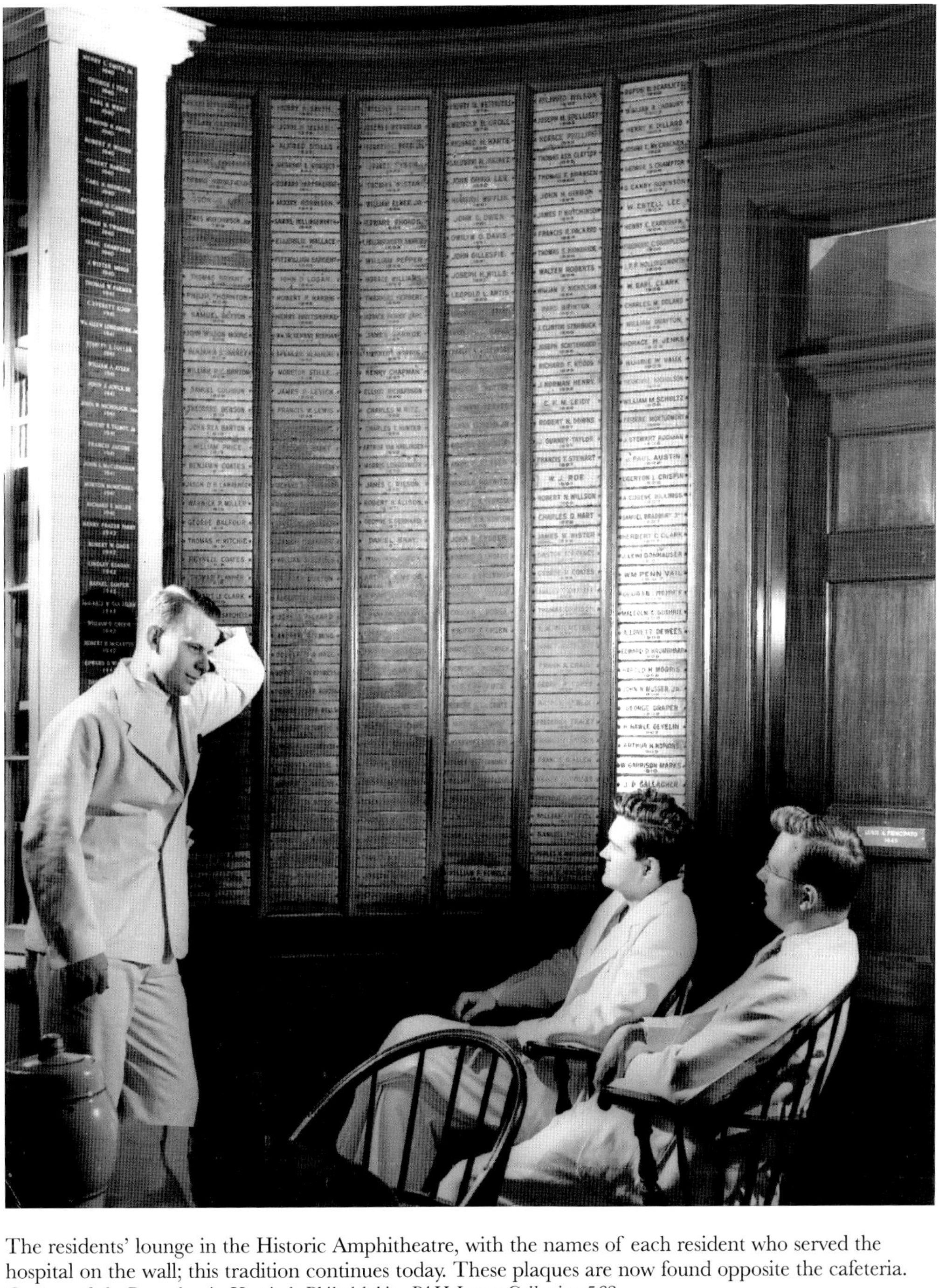

The residents' lounge in the Historic Amphitheatre, with the names of each resident who served the hospital on the wall; this tradition continues today. These plaques are now found opposite the cafeteria. *Courtesy of the Pennsylvania Hospital, Philadelphia, PAH Image Collection 563.*

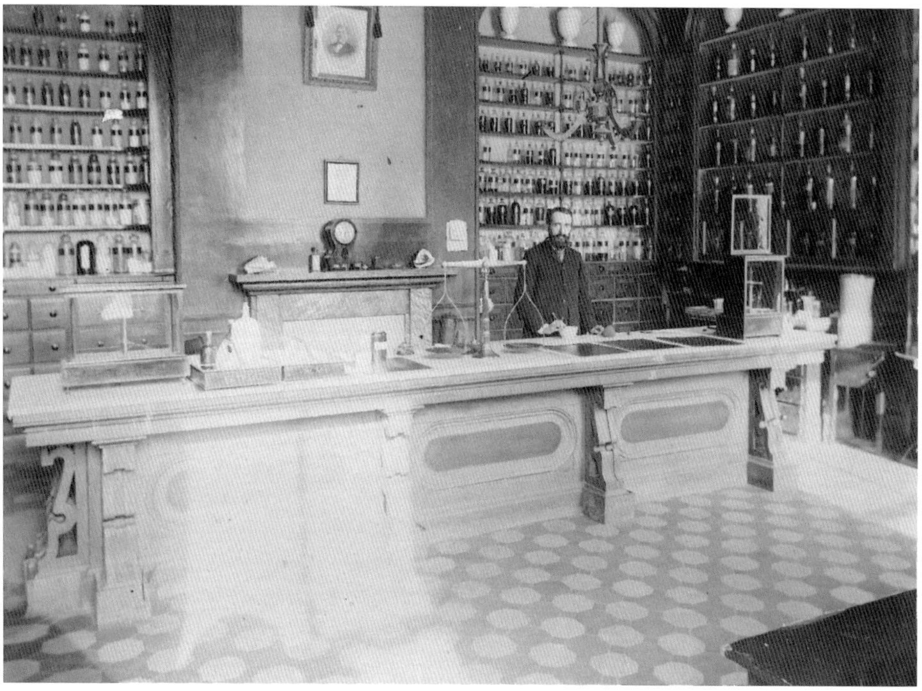

A late nineteenth-century image of the apothecary; this room is now the Great Court Conference Room. *Courtesy of the Pennsylvania Hospital, Philadelphia, PAH Image Collection.*

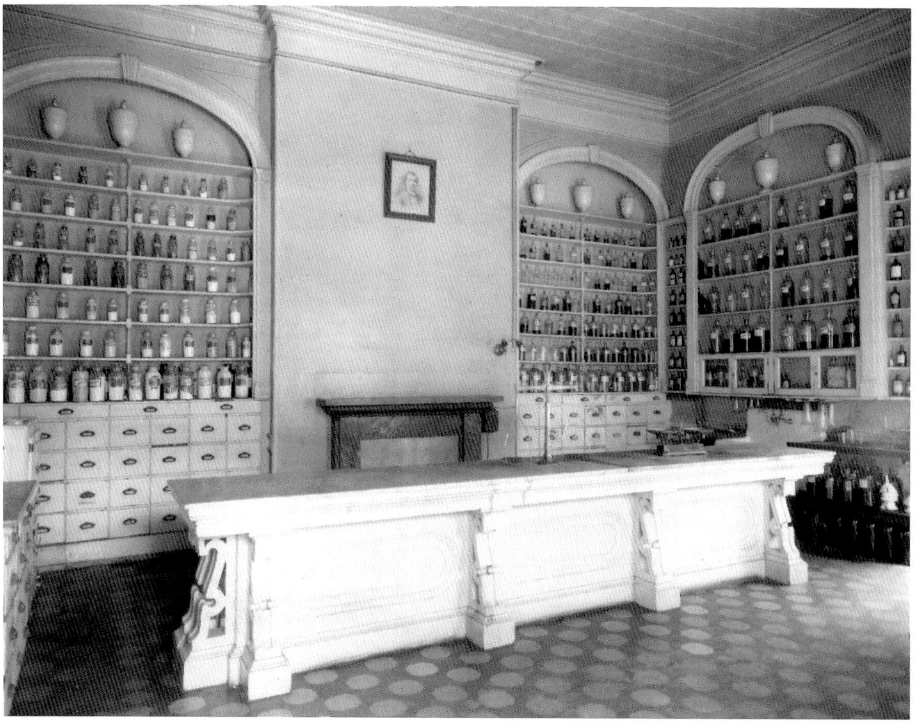

A 1927 image of the apothecary. *Courtesy of the Pennsylvania Hospital, Philadelphia, PAH Image Collection.*

the first floor. If you look closely among the rows and rows of small plaques, you will find one from 1941 inscribed with the name of "C. Everett Koop," onetime surgeon general of the United States.

As for Ehrenzeller, he used his certificate from the hospital to work as an assistant surgeon during the Revolutionary War. After the war, he served as a doctor in the small towns of West Chester and Goshen, again earning distinction as one of the few nineteenth-century "village physicians" who were able to support themselves without having to resort to a second occupation.[29]

ADMISSIONS IN THE COLONIAL PERIOD: DAILY ROUTINE

Pennsylvania Hospital's founders created the facility to serve the sick poor, but the managers needed a mix of paying and nonpaying patients to keep the operation afloat. Keeping in mind their mission, nonpaying patients greatly outnumbered paying patients in the colonial years. In 1774, when the hospital was doing well financially with an income of £1,264, there was just enough money to support seventy free beds. Still, over a hundred charity cases were accepted, with the managers diverting donations away from the capital stock and directly into caring for these needy citizens.

Some patients still had to be turned away, though. (There are no records on the number of sick poor who applied for admission.) Patients who paid for their care were charged ten shillings per week, a cost that did not allow the hospital to break even. Once the new building was completed, however, more patients could be admitted. Costs per patient took a dip as well. As a result, the hospital earned almost three shillings a week per paying patient, meaning that for every three paying patients, one patient could be admitted at no charge.

African American patients were admitted to the hospital, some as free persons who qualified as poor patients, and some as slaves. Initially, slaves were admitted as regular paying patients, with their masters expected to cover the cost of their care. In 1761,

> *it being observed that several Negro slaves have been taken into the House as pay patients at a rate lower than we think can be afforded, it is unanimously agreed that none be hereafter received at less than fifteen shillings per week and as much as the sitting managers shall think the circumstances of the case may require.*

The managers' explanation—that the hospital could not afford to charge less than fifteen shillings per week—is puzzling because the average weekly per-patient cost was under ten shillings. It is possible that the largely Quaker managers charged slaves' masters a premium because the managers objected to slavery. The board, for instance, made note of its concern for a free black man's security. When George Saunders, a "boy with a round in his arm by an engagement at sea," was admitted, a man named Nicholas

Jones promised to pay burial expenses if he died. The managers noted that "care must be taken on his [Saunders's] discharge that N. Jones takes no advantage of him for his entertainment here."

Beginning in 1768, the managers also decided to charge a higher rate for paying patients afflicted with venereal disease. It was a fine line to walk—to refuse such patients would make the managers' sense of charity look suspect, but to welcome them might mean the hospital was condoning immoral behavior. The board took a middle ground: poor patients with venereal disease were treated gratis, as any other poor patient. Those in a position to pay were charged fifteen shillings a week.[30]

Patients who were physically able to do so were put to work at the hospital. In 1754, managers Isaac Jones and Evan Morgan decided to provide spinning wheels, wool and flax for patient use. On occasion, the hospital made the work instructional so that patients who were permanently disabled could attempt to support themselves after discharge. In 1760, the hospital set out to help a ten-year-old blind girl who had been a patient for some time. An ad was placed in the *Pennsylvania Gazette* in order to find someone who would "undertake to instruct her in such business as she may be capable of, to enable her to make a living."

Few details of the typical patient's day exist. Beds for the physically ill were lined up along two long walls of each of the two wards, with no mention of curtains separating patient space. A patient's day was regulated by the sun, with breakfast served early. Nurses and maids came around to empty bedpans, make beds, sweep floors and generally aid patients. Patients who were able to move around also assisted other patients. Two days a week, doctors and their apprentices made rounds. Lunch was served at noon, and during the afternoon, patients received visitors and read religious tracts that were on hand if they were literate. The routine was decidedly dull—many patients could not read and had no visitors. The evening meal was early, and then the lights went out. By 1762, patient misconduct caused the board to order "a sufficient number of the rules of conduct to be observed by the patients to be hung up in the several wards."[31]

Patients were fed a limited diet, suggesting that it was not thought desirable for the ill to eat large meals. According to one diet bill from 1759, patients would be served a pint of coffee or a pint of broth for breakfast; eight ounces of boiled mutton or veal for the midday meal, dinner; and mush with sugar or butter for supper, the late meal. The diet varied a little—water gruel might be served, or rice milk, or "a baked Indian pudding." The managers noted that "Potatoes & Turnips are occasionally to be added."[32]

From the early patient records, some interesting cases stand out. On October 9, 1754, "a French deserter afflicted with Remittent Fever" was admitted. On March 31, 1756, "Admitted, a poor Patient from Berks County, having a Gunshot wound and fractured Bone in one Arm done by the 6th inst. by the Enemy Indians, James Biddle of said County Security." On May 6, 1756, "patient, being cured, marched off on the 17th instant, without being regularly dismissed." On October 3, 1764, "Admitted, a poor patient, with Disiness in the Head having been much abused by Indians." One man was not a cooperative patient, and he was discharged on November 27, 1758, "for refusing to submit to the advice of Physicians." Some patients cause the modern reader puzzlement: on July 30, 1764, "Admitted a poor Patient hurt of drinking cold Water."[33]

THE HOSPITAL DURING THE REVOLUTION

In June 1775, the managers first made mention of the American Revolution, noting that "the present state of public affairs will not permit" the importation of more drugs to the hospital.[34] Despite the pacifist roots of its mostly Quaker founders, records show that the hospital was resolute in its decision to care for the country's soldiers, with the first wounded admitted in July 1776.[35] Though it severely tested the hospital and its managers, it did bolster a flagging patient census—a month earlier, the hospital had been running at just 50 percent of its capacity.

In December, the Pennsylvania Council of Safety ordered that the hospital be used to treat sick and injured soldiers of the Continental army. Fifty soldiers were admitted on December 5, 1776. The balance of patients began to shift as more soldiers—Continental and captured Hessians—than civilians were being treated. Dr. Thomas Bond, who was responsible for the injured and sick soldiers, promised to pay for their medications.

Though the hospital received some payment for its care, it was not enough, and soon the hospital was in financial trouble. The inflation that was plaguing Philadelphia forced the hospital to increase its charge for paying patients from ten to fifteen shillings per week. Soon after, the managers decided to pay off hospital bills using Continental currency, which was fast depreciating. By the spring of 1777, most of the American soldiers had left the hospital. But that August, British General Howe began to move toward Philadelphia. Howe and his troops edged Washington out of the city, and by September, Philadelphia was occupied by the Redcoats.

On September 26, "a great number of sick and wounded soldiers (without previous notice given, or application to the Managers) were brought into the hospital." Chaos ensued after the hospital's takeover; the British soldiers made it difficult to keep order and to treat civilian patients. Managers admitted that the quality of patient care had declined, and even the quality of the food they could serve to the patients was poorer during that bitterly cold, calamitous winter, when Washington and his men camped at Valley Forge. (A "diet bill" in the manager's minutes from that era, however, still notes that the patients were routinely fed portions including half a pound of beef, half a pound of potatoes and parsnips and a pint of beer for supper.) The managers had to borrow money to keep the hospital afloat after the British outlawed the use of Revolutionary currency.[36]

In March 1778, King George III ordered the evacuation of Philadelphia, and British soldiers never returned to the city. The hospital still suffered. Four of the managers had to flee the city as part of a party of mostly Quaker men forced out because of supposed Tory sympathies. Prices for staples necessary to run a hospital were at wartime highs. To combat some of its problems during that year, the managers attempted to come up with creative ways of running the hospital. In August 1778, "in consideration of the present high price of milk," the managers purchased three cows; in December of that year, the board, "taking into consideration the urgent want of blankets" formed a committee to procure an immediate supply. The managers even considered "discharging" the steward and the matron to cut costs.[37]

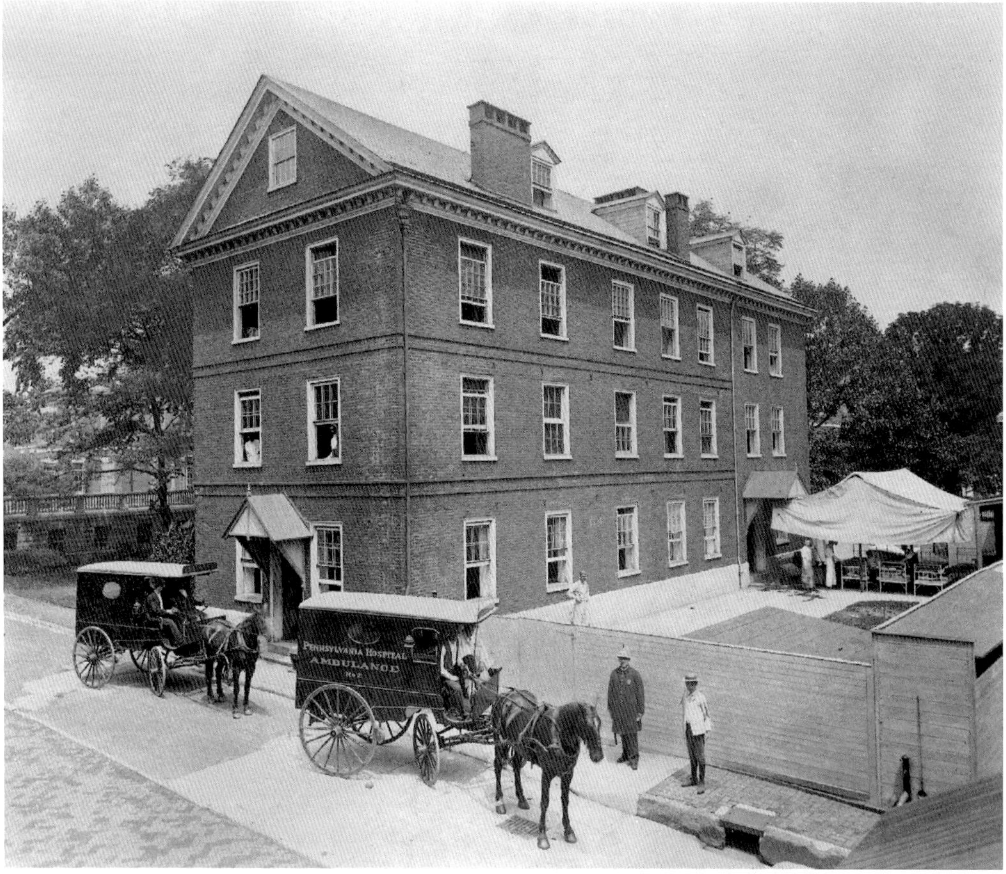

An 1895 image of the Elaboratory. Notice the tent set up to care for patients in the heat of the summer, as well as the horse-drawn ambulances. *Courtesy of the Pennsylvania Hospital, Philadelphia, PAH Image Collection 2620a.*

During this period, more Continental soldiers were admitted to the hospital—this time subject to the same rules as private patients—and the hospital agreed to rent out the "Elaboratory," a two-story building detached from the hospital and previously used by the apothecary for mixing drugs.[38] The assembly looked favorably upon Pennsylvania Hospital's efforts, awarding it the seemingly princely sum of 10,000 of Continental money, but in reality, this added up to only about £163 sterling. Still, the assembly granted the hospital all unclaimed shares from prizes taken by privateers; it also gave the hospital the revenue from fines imposed upon its members.[39]

The years after the Revolution were a time of recovery for the battered hospital. In 1779, one manager wrote of the "very languishing state" of the hospital, and of his fear that it "can not long be supported." The managers set about fundraising—they published abstracts of accounts of the hospital, slashed salaries and reduced the amount of liquor served to patients. Newspaper articles solicited funds from the public, British friends were called upon and benefit concerts and lectures helped to bolster finances. So did a new program of investing in rental properties. Gradually, the financial ship was righted, and the hospital began a period of expansion, with both the West Wing (1796) and center structure of the hospital built by 1804, as envisioned in the original design of the building.[40]

YELLOW FEVER EPIDEMIC

In 1793, a yellow fever epidemic swept Philadelphia. It was noted by the managers that "a very malignant disorder, commonly called the Yellow Fever, hath raged with great Violence. In 99 days upwards of four thousand persons have died in the city and liberties."[41] City authorities had set up a special hospital specifically for those suffering from the disease, and the managers, unaware that the disease was spread by mosquito and not human contact, resolved to keep their hospital free from infection. However, Dr. John Foulke, a physician on staff, admitted two patients suffering from yellow fever to the hospital. When the managers learned of his error, they ordered Dr. Foulke "to visit the patients and investigate the matter, and do everything in his power to prevent the increase of the disease."

Soon after, the managers suspended their monthly meetings because of the epidemic. Many moneyed physicians (including Dr. Foulke) were fleeing the city, but some of the hospital's doctors—notably, Dr. Benjamin Rush, Dr. Philip Syng Physick and Dr. Caspar Wistar—remained in the city and at work. Dr. Rush was particularly active in treating yellow fever cases, going to homes around the city and bloodletting and purging patients. He contracted yellow fever twice and lost three apprentices to the disease.[42] The managers' hiatus lasted four months, but although the hospital staff was relatively unharmed, roughly 10 percent of the city's population fell victim to the epidemic. In subsequent yellow fever outbreaks at the end of the eighteenth century, the hospital continued its policy of excluding patients suffering from the disease.[43]

CHANGING ADMISSIONS POLICIES

By 1796, the cash-strapped managers had adopted a policy of limiting charity cases. The rule was that no more than thirty nonpaying patients could live at the hospital at once, although emergency cases could occasionally be admitted. Two years later, the managers attempted to have the burial guarantee stricken. But the hospital charter stated that the board would have to receive approval from the contributors and some state officials for such a change, and the managers failed to obtain the necessary approvals. By 1803, burial security had reached five dollars per person.

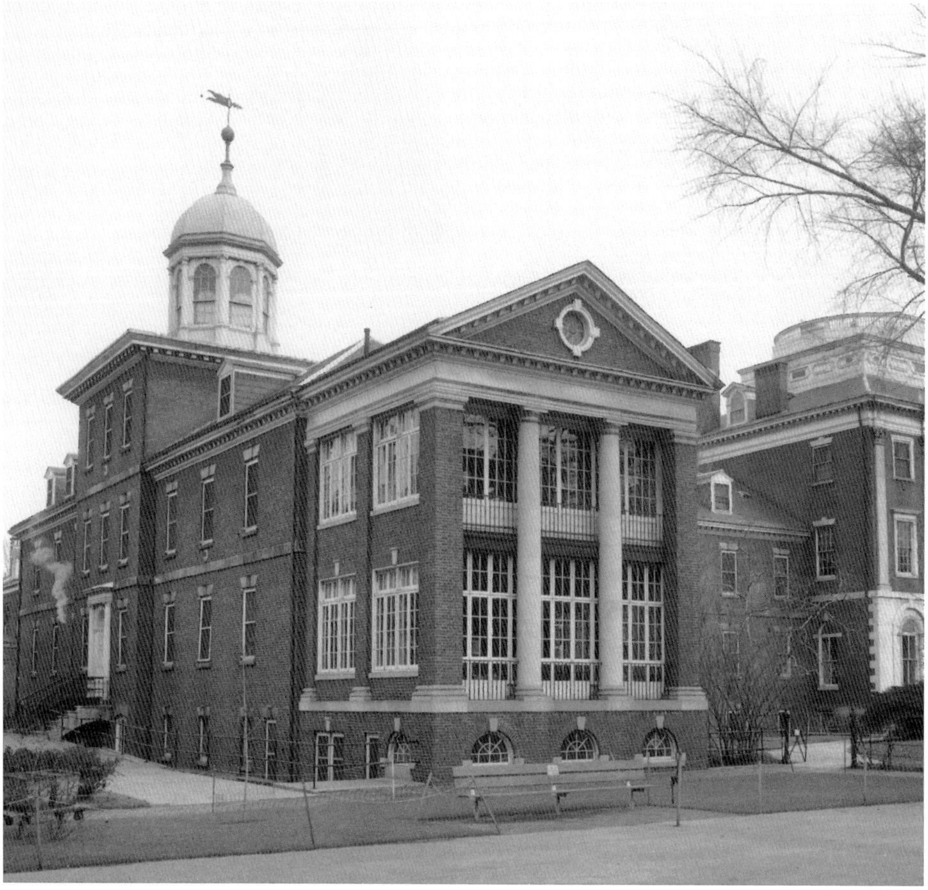

A 1950s view of the West Wing Pine Building. The area that is roped off is the current site of the Physic Garden. *Courtesy of the Pennsylvania Hospital, Philadelphia, PAH Image Collection.*

PSYCHIATRY

From the hospital's earliest days, caring for the "distemper'd in mind" was an important part of its mission. Benjamin Franklin and Thomas Bond certainly were concerned by the increasing number of "lunaticks" wandering the streets of their growing city, and it follows that four of the first six patients admitted were psychiatric patients. During the colonial period, psychiatric patients occupied about one-third of Pennsylvania Hospital's beds; after the American Revolution, that figure rose to about one-half. In fact, Pennsylvania Hospital is considered the birthplace of American psychiatry, thanks to the innovative Dr. Benjamin Rush.

Conditions for the insane, however, were initially quite poor. The mentally ill were housed in the basement in cells "damp and unwholesome," with plank floors "arched

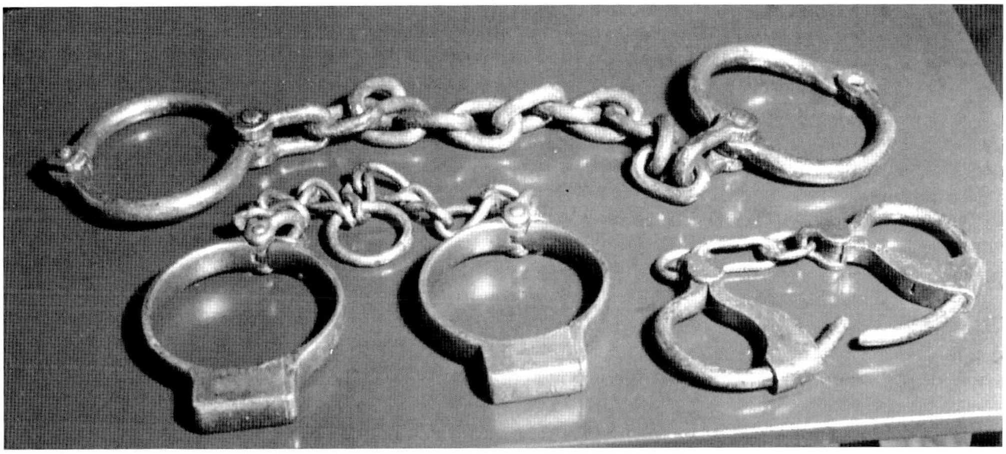

An image of the restraint chains used in the eighteenth and early nineteenth centuries for mentally ill patients at the Pennsylvania Hospital. *Courtesy of the Pennsylvania Hospital, Philadelphia, PAH Image Collection 1672.*

below to prevent dampness and preclude association with rats." The wards smelled bad; Dr. Rush complained of the noxious odors from the chamber pots used in the cells as late as 1810. A number of patients died of pulmonary disease. The care they received was considered humane at the time, but the cells were still quite cold and uncomfortable, and patients were often restrained in hand irons, leg locks and "mad-shirts" (straitjackets).[44]

Still, escaping patients were a problem. In 1758, two male patients managed to part the iron bars of their cells and escape seven times. Prompted by their repeated fleeing, the board brought a blacksmith in to strengthen the bars. Another patient's escape was quite complex—he bored through the door of his cell and forced out the staples of the iron bolts. In 1773, seven "elopements" were recorded in August alone.[45] Wealthier patients paid a premium—ten dollars per week—for better care than that received by the average insane patient. A private servant was sometimes included in that charge, and separate quarters were always part of the package.

The insane, many of whom were violent, were seen as curiosities, and peering at them through the iron bars was a popular pastime. At first, the managers had a fence erected "in order to prevent the disturbance which is given to the lunatics confined in their cells by the great numbers of people who frequently resort and converse with them." The fence proved inadequate to keep out the curious, and so in 1763, the board had a "hatch door" constructed. The inscription gave notice that those wishing to view the insane should pay four pence at least to offset "the great crowds who resort here of late, giving trouble and disturbance."[46]

Curious visitors were sometimes problematic. In 1784, hospital physicians "recommended that some regulations may be made in respect to persons visiting the Hospital, particularly in adopting such rules as would tend to prevent the lunatic patients from being interrupted and disturbed in their course of medication." In response, the board adopted its own rule that no more than two persons at once "be permitted to go into the cells and those persons to be attended by the cell keeper, and not suffered to speak to such patients."[47]

Though the hospital's treatment of the mentally ill seems far from ideal by our modern standard, the idea that such patients should be cared for at all was rather revolutionary. Most colonial Americans believed that the insane were subhuman and should be relegated to poorhouses or jail cells without any care at all.[48] As the colonies entered into the American Revolution, numbers of insane patients began to increase sharply. By the end of the war, in fact, the nature of the hospital had shifted dramatically.

During the colonial period, restrictions were put in place on the number of insane patients; Pennsylvania Hospital was mostly a general hospital. By 1783, the final year of the war, and until the end of the century, the hospital was in many ways an insane asylum. More than half of the resident patients were mentally ill. In some ways, this helped boost the hospital's financial situation. Most physically ill patients came from poor families and were unable to pay for a hospital stay. But mentally ill patients often came from wealthy families with the means to fund a stay. While there is no record of a decision to favor applications of mentally ill patients, especially those who could pay, the numbers seem to indicate that one was made. In 1780, the board wrote John Fothergill "that we have been under the sad necessity of refusing many proper objects of our charity."[49]

By the beginning of the nineteenth century, Dr. Benjamin Rush, who had joined the hospital's staff in 1783, began to revolutionize the treatment of psychiatric patients. Dr. Rush, who is called the "Father of American Psychiatry," was a signer of the Declaration of Independence. He believed that mental illness was a disease of the mind, rather than possession by demons, moonbeams, celibacy or tobacco use, as had previously been believed. He understood that mental patients should be treated humanely, and his "tranquilizing chair"—a new way of confining patients, it reduced the flow of blood

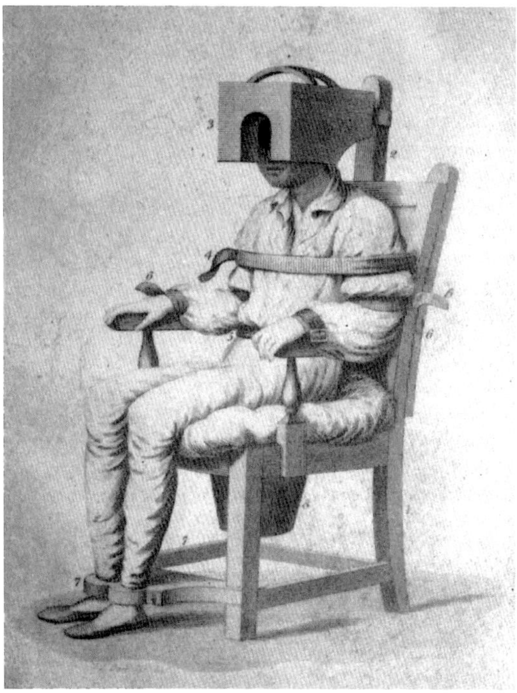

Benjamin Rush's tranquilizing chair was supposed to control the flow of blood toward the brain, and by lessening muscular action or reducing motor activity, it reduced the force and frequency of the pulse. *Courtesy of the Pennsylvania Hospital, Philadelphia, PAH Image Collection.*

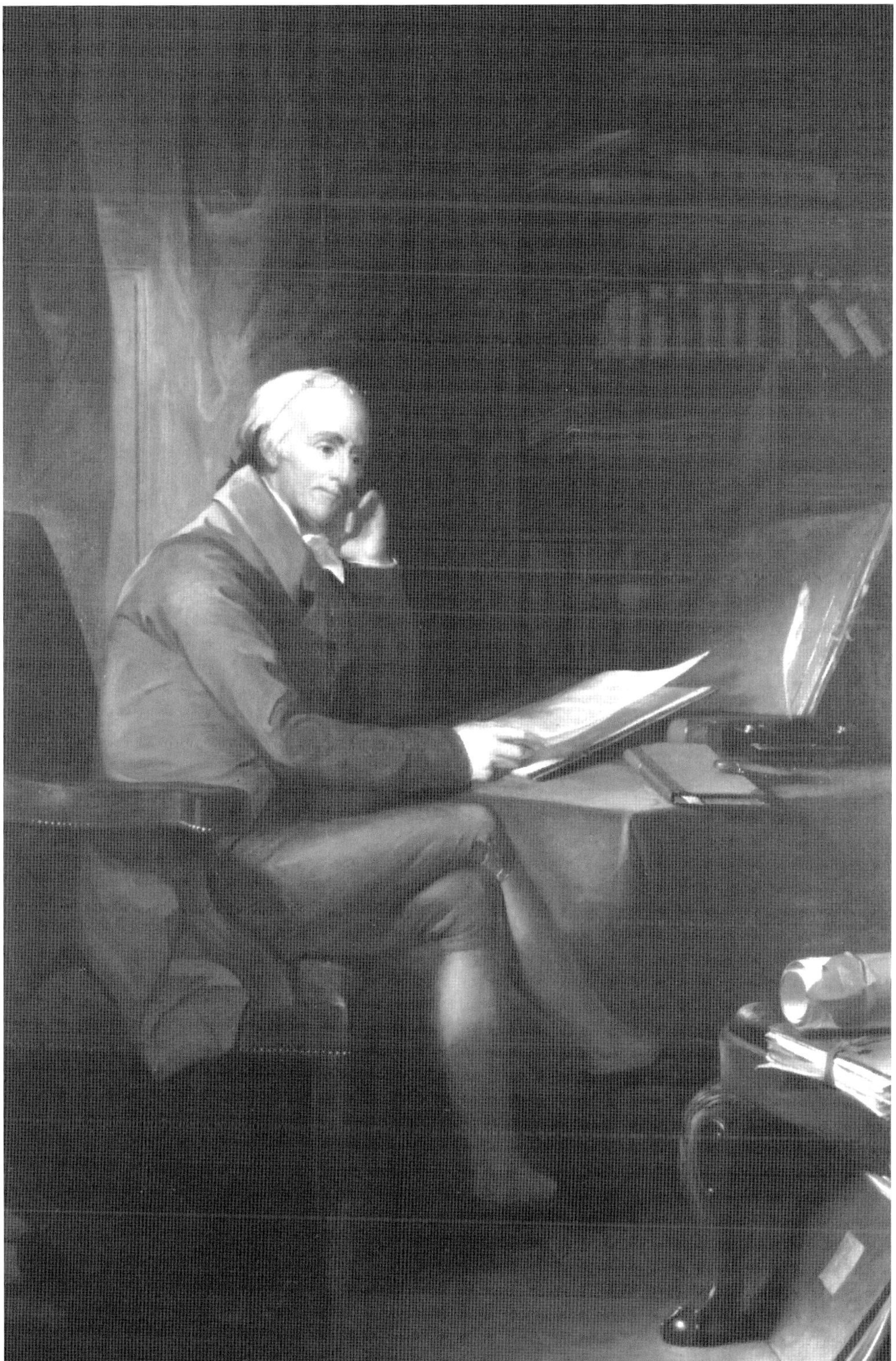

A Thomas Sully portrait of Dr. Benjamin Rush (1813). The painting is on display outside the Historic Library. *Courtesy of the Pennsylvania Hospital, Philadelphia, PAH Image Collection.*

to the brain by binding the limbs—was a better alternative than a straitjacket.[50] (Rush believed that insanity could be caused by disappointed love, excessive drinking, lead poisoning, measles or religious fervor. Among his favored treatments were bloodletting and purging.) Still, Dr. Rush urged the hospital to halt its policy of chaining the most seriously mentally ill in unheated cells in the basement, and he stopped Philadelphians from coming to the hospital to view patients as a form of entertainment.

Dr. Rush was an early believer in what is now called occupational therapy. In 1798, he suggested that "certain employments be devised for such of the deranged people as are capable of working." He proposed spinning, sewing and churning for the female patients, and for the men, gardening, grinding corn for the hospital's horse and cows and cutting straw.[51] Under Dr. Rush's guidance, the hospital's reputation grew, and the number of insane patients, who often stayed for extended periods of time, far exceeded the number of physically ill patients. Dr. Rush was a well-respected scholar and author; his two most noted works were *Observations on Yellow Fever* (1762) and *Observations and Inquiries Upon the Diseases of the Mind* (1812), the first psychiatric textbook printed in the country.[52]

Many notable and colorful patients passed through Pennsylvania Hospital's doors during this era. The case of the "lunatic hermit" attracted attention throughout the city. The patient, "a remarkably neat and tidy Sailor," was admitted in 1765 and lived briefly in the cells, proving troublesome, quarreling with patients and employees. But then the patient escaped the cells and fled to the cupola of the East Wing, where he fended off all attempts to remove him. Finally, the staff gave up and simply put bedding there. The patient, who was known for his long nails and matted beard and hair, lived in the cupola until he died in 1774.[53]

Eventually, the hospital grew too crowded, and because the thinking of the day dictated that the mentally ill needed to be confined, the managers felt they ought to build new quarters for their mentally ill patients. In 1832, the managers resolved to create a separate asylum for the majority of the hospital's patients. A large farm, whose boundaries were Forty-fourth through Forty-ninth and Market Street and Haverford Road in what was then Philadelphia's western suburbs, was purchased from Matthew Arrison in 1835. (Three years later, the board purchased an additional 9.5 acres for "walking grounds" for the patients.) The Pennsylvania Hospital for the Insane rose there, based on a design by Isaac Holden, who had won an architectural competition sponsored by the managers.

The cornerstone for the new facility was laid on July 26, 1836. In the winter of 1841, one hundred mentally ill patients journeyed by carriage from the city center to their new outpost in the rural suburbs. The new asylum formally opened on January 1. The hospital sat on 101 acres, flanked by woods and meadows.[54] It featured stone arches and large parlors, and each patients' quarters had more sun, heat, plumbing and ventilation than the rooms of above-average homes in Philadelphia.[55] There was a deer park, a flower garden, a railroad built for patients' amusement and a Gentlemen's and a Ladies' Pleasure Grounds. The new superintendent, Dr. Thomas Story Kirkbride, and his family moved to the grounds as well, living in a mansion on-site that had been owned by Paul Busti, an area merchant.

Dr. Kirkbride, a Quaker, arrived to head the new hospital for the insane, and under his supervision, psychiatry again reached new heights. He adopted the new "moral

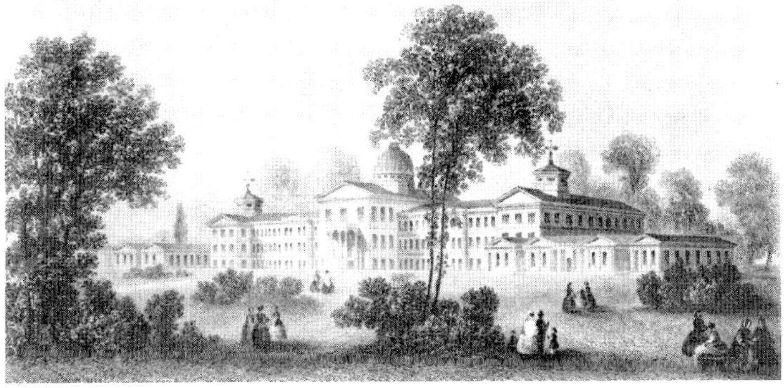

Pennsylvania Hospital for the Insane Female Department. This image is a reproduction of an engraving by J.M. Butler (1860). *Courtesy of the Pennsylvania Hospital, Philadelphia, PAH Image Collection 48.*

treatment" first popular with European reformers. Dr. Kirkbride advocated kindness to patients, eliminating the use of restraints when possible, encouraging recreation and exercise and hiring attendants and nurses, not "keepers," of patients. He believed that greater freedom typically resulted in better behavior among patients, and he insisted on treating those at his hospital with dignity.[56] He asserted that patients "are not disabled from appreciating books…or enjoying many intellectual and physical comforts." In fact, the hospital was generally known as "Kirkbride's" in honor of him. Under Kirkbride's supervision, "evening entertainments" were held—lectures, choir performances or shows from what he called the "magic lantern," a slide projector that beamed hand-painted slides onto the wall. Topics ranged from history to religion to travel, and Kirkbride believed that the shows served as both therapy and entertainment. Patients could also browse the library or in-house museum.[57]

The new hospital was not the first free-standing psychiatric hospital in the United States, but it was the first to be affiliated with a general hospital. In 1844, Dr. Kirkbride gathered the superintendents of thirteen asylums in Philadelphia. They formed the Association of Medical Superintendents of American Institutions for the Insane, which later became the American Psychiatric Association. It was the first subspecialty medical association, and Pennsylvania Hospital would eventually boast twelve presidents of the organization, more than any other hospital in the country. The fourteen leaders of Kirkbride's group remained close, and that group eventually became known as the Ivy League Private Practice Hospital group, which continues today. Later, in 1854, Kirkbride wrote *On the Construction, Organization and General Arrangements of Hospitals for the Insane*, which came to be known as "the Kirkbride Plan." It was widely accepted and implemented in hospitals throughout the country.

The institution continued to thrive under Kirkbride's supervision; its population boomed, and though additions had been made to the original building, the need for a new, separate facility was soon evident. On July 7, 1856, the cornerstone for a new building was laid. This new building would rise at Forty-ninth and Market Streets, five blocks west of the original structure, and was built with money from private contributions. The new structure was set aside for male patients and was known as the Department for Males. The original building became the Department for Females.

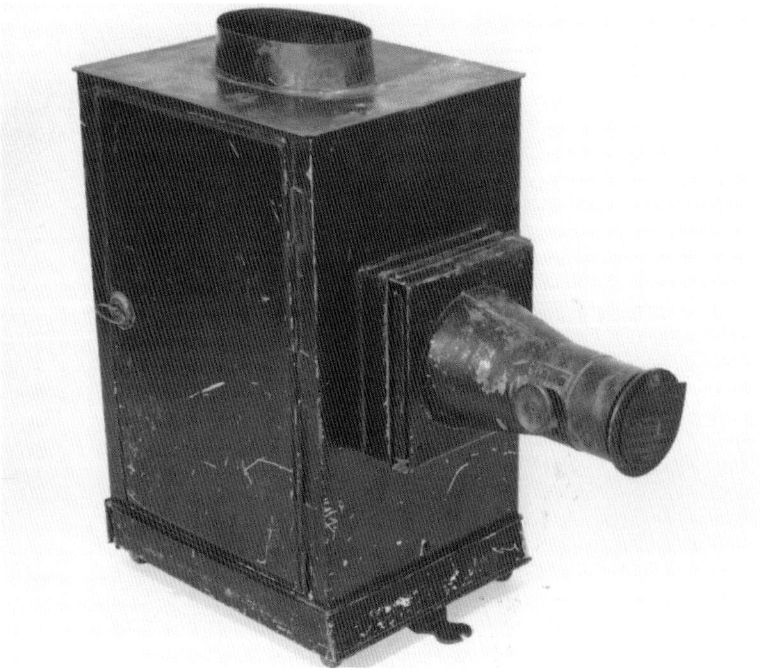

The "Magic Lantern" was used by Dr. Kirkbride as entertainment for the Institute patients. They would gather in the auditorium and watch slide shows of travelogues, among other entertaining images. *Courtesy of the Pennsylvania Hospital, Philadelphia, PAH Image Collection 1658.1.*

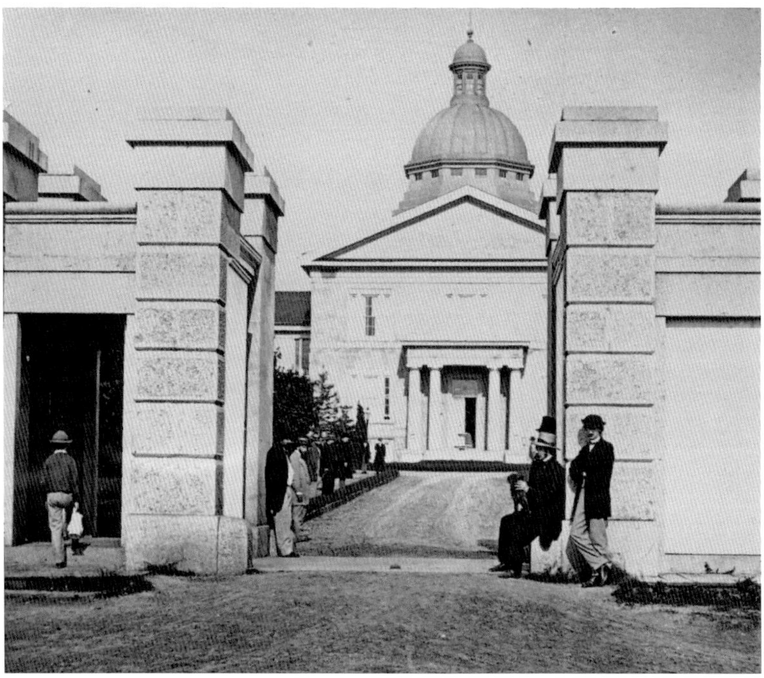

Front entrance to Forty-fourth Street, Institute Building (1870). *Courtesy of the Pennsylvania Hospital, Philadelphia, PAH Image Collection.*

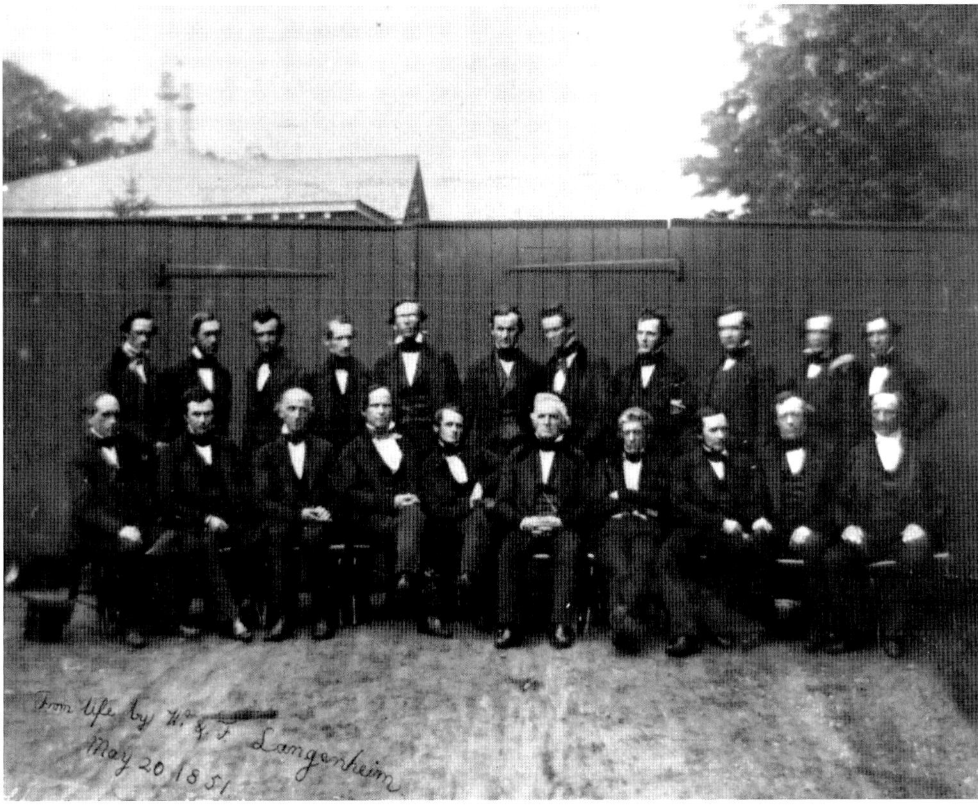

The earliest known image of an annual meeting of the Association of Medical Superintendents of Institutions for the Insane, which later become the American Psychiatric Association, on the grounds of the Institute of Pennsylvania Hospital in 1851. *Courtesy of the Pennsylvania Hospital, Philadelphia, PAH Image Collection.*

Kirkbride oversaw the hospital until his death in 1883. Dr. John B. Chapin succeeded him, followed by Dr. Owen Copp, whose chief contribution to the institution was the School of Nursing for Men (see page 81 for details). Under Dr. Copp's stewardship, the organization officially became known as the Department of Mental and Nervous Diseases in 1918. Shortly thereafter, two young doctors began to make their marks—Dr. Earl Bond, who became physician in chief in 1922, and Dr. Edward A. Strecker, who was tapped to head a new outpatient service at Forty-ninth Street.[58] It was the hospital's first outpatient service for the mentally ill, opened for those who needed psychiatric care, but for whom constant hospital supervision was unnecessary. The new service proved popular, so in 1930, male inpatients were transferred back to the Forty-fourth Street facility so the Forty-ninth Street property could be the center of outpatient operations. The Forty-ninth Street facility was called the Institute for Mental Hygiene of the Pennsylvania Hospital or, more commonly, the Institute.

Most outpatients suffered from ordinary neuroses. "Some of the commoner problems," it was written at the time, "were sleeplessness, fatigue, depression, feelings of inferiority, and differences in getting on with people. The patients have been decidedly above the average in intelligence and other gifts."[59] Drs. Bond and Strecker, together with Dr. Kenneth Appel, who came to the hospital in 1929, favored breaking down distinctions between a person who was mentally ill and one who was not. In many ways, the trio helped lift traditional taboos that surrounded psychiatry. A 1947 *Saturday Evening Post* article featured Dr. Strecker, proclaiming that "He Made Psychiatry Respectable."[60]

Dr. Strecker proved an innovative, cutting-edge psychiatrist, and during World Wars I and II he was considered the world's foremost authority on shellshock.[61] He was one of the first physicians to recognize alcoholism as a mental illness rather than a moral failing. In 1935, Pennsylvania Hospital's psychiatric arm was the first institution to hire a recovering person as an addiction counselor. Together, Dr. Strecker and Francis Chambers Jr., a recovering alcoholic patient, developed the "dual therapy" approach for alcoholics—a method that combined abstinence and psychological counseling. The substance abuse unit was renamed "the Strecker Program" in Dr. Strecker's honor, and in 1989 it was named "Treatment Center of the Year" by the American Council on Alcoholism.[62] It was under Dr. Strecker's supervision that the Forty-ninth Street property was renamed the Institute. The Institute was one of the few hospital programs nationally that treated both the severely mentally ill and those who needed help coping with stresses of everyday life.

Dr. Joseph Hughes joined the Institute in 1934, at a time when insulin and other chemically induced shock therapies were being used to treat many mental disorders. These were considered hazardous procedures, but at the time, no other methods existed to treat those who did not respond to psychotherapy, occupational therapy or the few medications that were used then. Hughes was fascinated by the work of two Italian physicians who were using electroshock therapy—changing the chemical balance of patients' brains. Dr. Hughes began experimenting with it in 1940 and built his own apparatus. The result was a model for future electroshock therapy units. As the pendulum swung away from using electroshock therapy, Dr. Hughes acknowledged the treatment was controversial, but he said it was never used unduly at the Institute.[63]

In 1959, the whole West Philadelphia campus became known as the Institute of the Pennsylvania Hospital. The Forty-fourth Street property was shuttered when the City of Philadelphia exercised its right of eminent domain to make way for a new subway project, and all patients were moved to the Forty-ninth Street property, where a new five-story "North Building" was opened to house them. Soon this building became the site of the region's first inpatient treatment center for adolescents.

The Hall-Mercer Community Mental Health & Mental Retardation Center opened in 1965. For years, inpatient care was still the standard, except in rare cases, but concern over conditions in state-run institutions was growing. New medications also allowed many mentally ill men and women who otherwise would have been forced to spend their lives in facilities to live in the community. In short, when it was possible to care for the mentally ill outside an inpatient setting, the preference was to do so, and Hall-Mercer and other community- and social-based outpatient programs grew out of that. To this day, Hall-Mercer (now located at 245 South Eighth Street) offers ongoing, personalized assistance, focusing on the neediest in the community—the homeless, patients suffering from AIDS, the elderly, developmentally disabled individuals, Asian Americans suffering from mental illness and children born to drug-addicted mothers.[64]

In 1971, the Mill Creek School was founded as part of the Institute's Adolescent Treatment program. A coeducational school licensed by the state, the school was originally known as the High School of the Institute of Pennsylvania Hospital. It was renamed in February 1972. Originally, the school was considered more therapeutic than academic—teachers placed more emphasis on learning as an activity than on what was actually being learned. When the school was renamed, however, the philosophy shifted, with academics coming to the forefront. Mill Creek was designed to mirror a typical high school in many ways. Grades, though, did not exist; students either passed or failed courses. Teachers were "young and able to relate to their students. They provide a warm and informal atmosphere for learning," a member of the hospital staff wrote at the time.[65] Today, the school remains a place for students who find it difficult to succeed in traditional classroom settings. Those who find hope at Mill Creek often have avoidant behavior, self-destructive thoughts or actions, problems with authority or substance abuse issues. The school prides itself on its peaceful, supportive atmosphere, and graduates often go on to succeed in other learning environments.[66] The Institute opened the region's first inpatient units for young adults in 1974 and inpatient units for eating disorders in 1986.[67]

In 1997, the Institute was closed, a casualty of declining payments from insurance companies and less demand for inpatient psychiatric services. The buildings were sold to CoreCare Systems Inc., and the hospital's behavioral health programs returned to their original location at Eighth and Spruce. Inpatient psychiatric care is now joined with the community mental health services offered by the Hall-Mercer Community Mental Health and Mental Retardation Center. These cutting-edge programs, plus the hospital's psychiatry and psychology teaching programs combined with the resources of the University of Pennsylvania Health System added with the merger in 1997, have expanded psychiatric services to a new level. In 2008, the inpatient psychiatric unit at the Hospital of the University of Pennsylvania was relocated to Pennsylvania Hospital, centralizing inpatient behavioral health in one spot.

MEDICAL LIBRARY AND HISTORIC COLLECTIONS

One of Pennsylvania Hospital's richest resources, the hospital's Historic Medical Library, began as a result of the contributions of two friends of Benjamin Franklin. Its first book came from Dr. John Fothergill on July 27, 1762. Fothergill sent the hospital a volume entitled *An Experimental History of the Materia Medica*, which, he said, was for the purpose of educating "Young Men of Physic." Thus began the first medical library in the country.

Fothergill's donation launched the library in earnest—purchases, bequests and other donations would soon cause the collection to grow. In 1763, staff physicians requested that student admissions fees to clinical lectures be used toward the purchase of books for the library. In 1767, forty-three volumes were received from Dr. Lloyd Zachary's estate, and fifty-five medical classics from the estate of Dr. Benjamin Morris. In 1775, Dr. John Coakley Lettsom, another friend to Franklin, was appointed agent for acquiring books in London. Dr. Lettsom purchased multiple medical texts from noted London bookseller William Strahan, who was immortalized by the Scottish writer James Boswell. Boswell also contributed additional money and books to the library.

Originally, the books were kept in the managers' meeting room in the East Wing, and in 1767, the managers paid five shillings to have a bookcase built in that space. Later, in 1804, the growing library moved with the managers to the center building into its present room. From about 1824 through 1835, the collection was moved to several different spots as the room it had occupied was used as the Lying-in Department. But by 1835, the room was again a library and it continues as such to this day.

The managers appointed a student to supervise the library, and very strict rules were put in place. Only managers, physicians and students were permitted to borrow books. The library was open one hour in the morning and one in the afternoon, twice a week. Borrowers were required to sign a promissory note to guarantee against damage

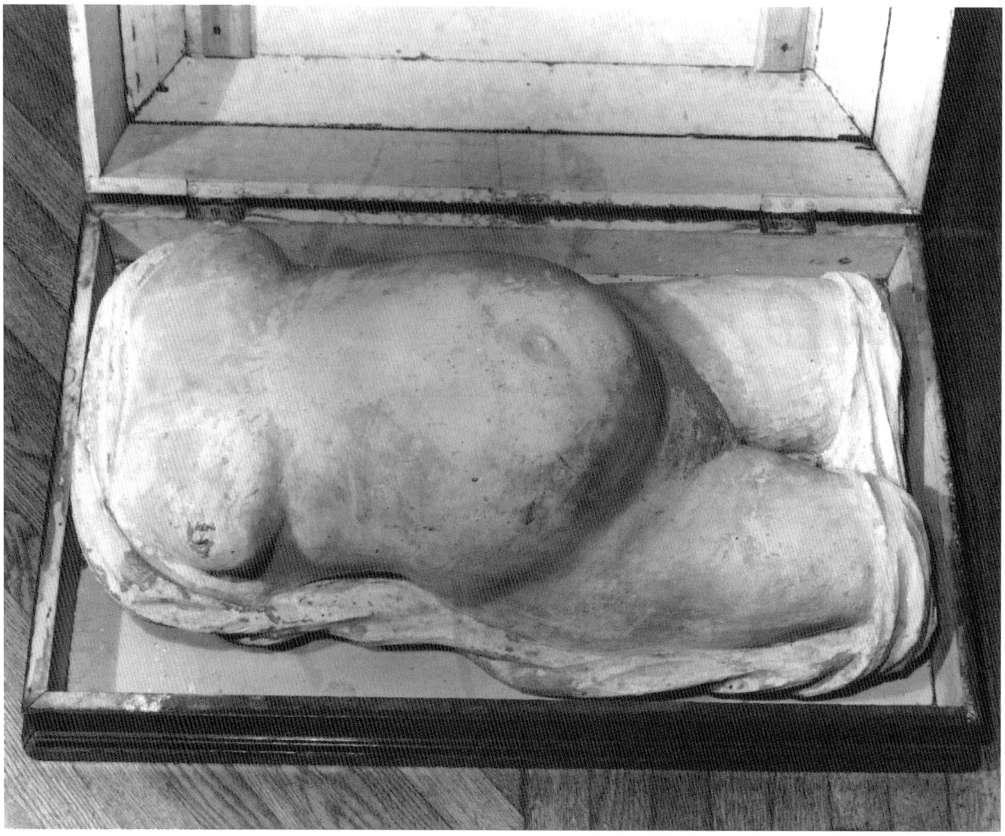

The first in a series of three obstetric plaster casts donated by Dr. John Fothergill to the Pennsylvania Hospital in 1762 for the "young men of physic." The cast was taken postmortem. *Courtesy of the Pennsylvania Hospital, Philadelphia, PAH Image Collection 1650a.*

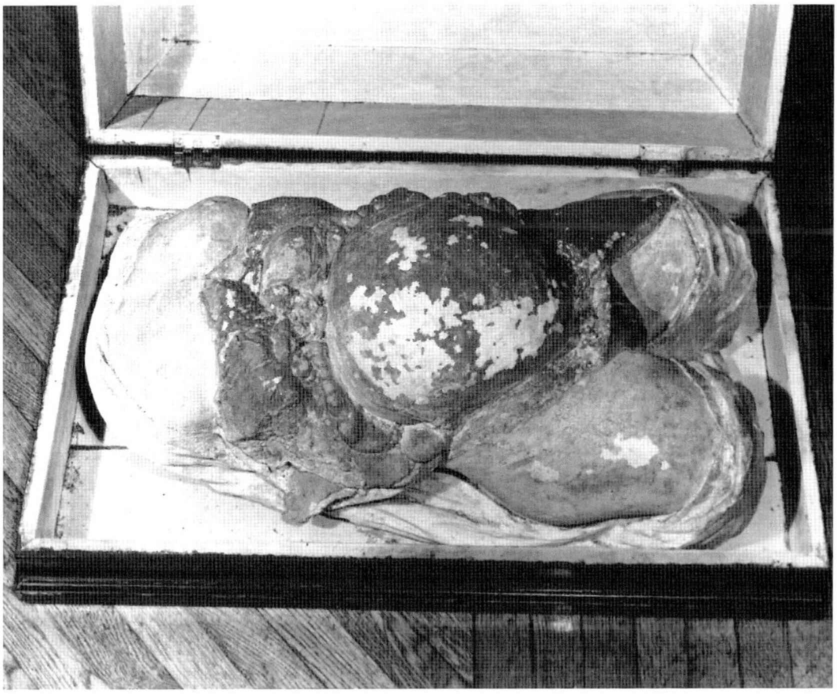

The second in a series of three obstetric plaster casts donated by Dr. John Fothergill. This view exposed the organs for student observation. *Courtesy of the Pennsylvania Hospital, Philadelphia, PAH Image Collection 1651a.*

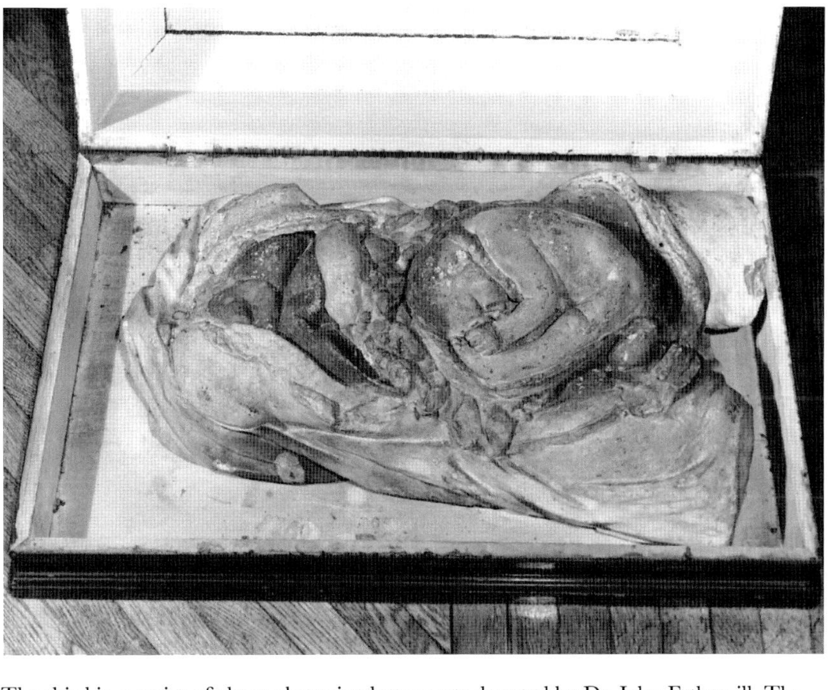

The third in a series of three obstetric plaster casts donated by Dr. John Fothergill. The final cast shows the fetus of the women in a breech position with the umbilical cord around the neck. *Courtesy of the Pennsylvania Hospital, Philadelphia, PAH Image Collection 1652b.*

or loss. Certain books, such as William Hunter's *Gravid Uterus* with illustrations by Jan Van Rymsdyk, could not be removed from the library. At the end of his one-year appointment, the student librarian had to account for each book and pay for any that were lost. Acquisitions were minimal during the Revolutionary War and subsequent budget crunch, but after Dr. Benjamin Rush complained that medical information in America was eight to ten years behind Europe, the managers moved to fix the problem. In 1790, when the first printed catalogue was prepared by Dr. Rush and Dr. Thomas Parke, the library had 366 volumes.

The collection grew in size and importance when the collection of William Byrd, of Westover, Virginia, one of the most noted book collectors in America, was donated to the hospital. His 3,625-volume library, which was known throughout the world, was sold to Isaac Zane, who kept them in Virginia until he sent them to his family to sell at auction in Philadelphia. There were rumors that Thomas Jefferson wanted to purchase some of the books, but deemed them too expensive. Zane died in 1795, and the books were sold piecemeal until 1800, when Zane's sister, Sarah, donated 124 medical and scientific volumes to Pennsylvania Hospital. It is believed that Pennsylvania Hospital has the largest portion of Byrd's collection.[68]

Another major addition came in 1817, when the managers purchased the library of Dr. Benjamin Smith Barton from his widow. Dr. Barton, a botanist, amassed a library of lovely volumes, including six volumes of Pierre Joseph Redoute's *Les Lilacees*, Mark Casteby's *Natural History of Carolina* and remarkable herbals of John Gerarde and Dr. Jacob Christoph Trew. Herbals were commonly used in colonial medicine, and these

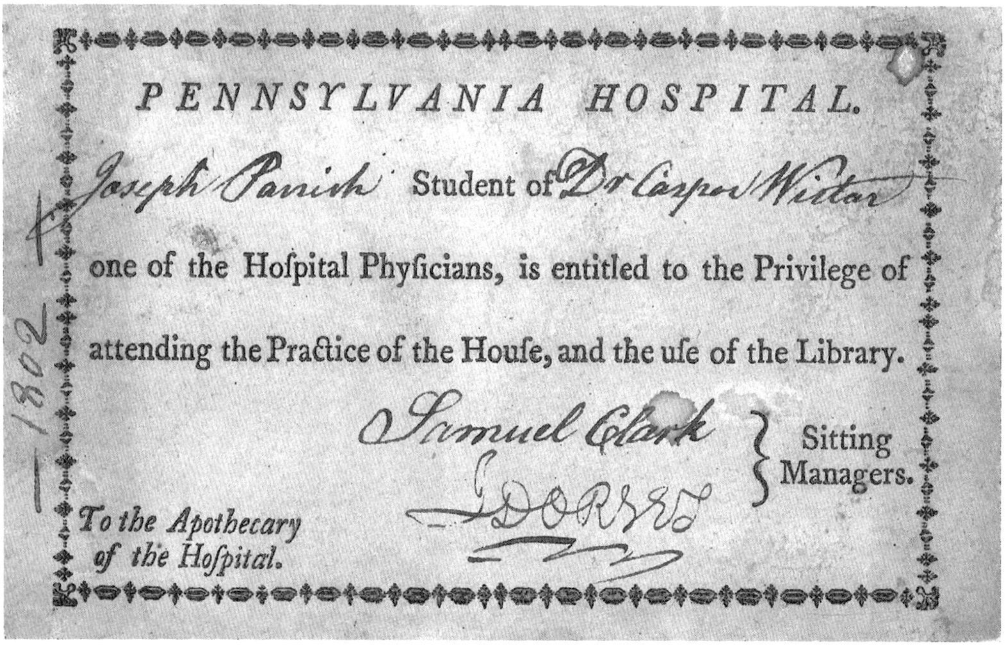
PENNSYLVANIA HOSPITAL.

Student of

one of the Hoſpital Phyſicians, is entitled to the Privilege of attending the Practice of the Houſe, and the uſe of the Library.

Sitting Managers.

To the Apothecary of the Hoſpital.

An admissions "ticket" used by students to attend lectures and use the library. This ticket was the property of Joseph Parrish, a medical student, under the guidance of Dr. Casper Wistar. *Courtesy of the Pennsylvania Hospital, Philadelphia, Administrative Records Collection.*

important works were valuable additions to the library.[69] The library continued to grow, and in 1847, the American Medical Association designated the library as the first, largest and most important medical library in the United States.

Two book lovers advanced the cause of the library. The first was William Gunn Malin, who began working at Pennsylvania Hospital in 1824 as a clerk. He later became the librarian, and under his supervision, the library acquired many of the 11 incunabula (books printed before 1501 in the earliest days of publishing) bound in 10 volumes. Malin also purchased subscriptions to important medical journals in multiple languages and had the sets bound. In 1829, Malin compiled a comprehensive catalog of the library's works, including the earlier 1790, 1794 and 1806 catalogs. About 150 volumes per year were purchased during his tenure. In 1840, Malin took over the hospital's newly opened psychiatric facility. He was no longer responsible for the library's day-to-day operations, but he remained an active advocate and supervised the library until his retirement in 1883.

Later in the hospital's history, Dr. Francis R. Packard did much for the library. He was intern, resident, staff physician, historian and honorary librarian from 1894 to 1950. His special concern for books led him to ask the board of managers to employ a librarian and prepare a card catalog to classify the library materials. He promoted the library among scholars and also wrote a history of the hospital, *Some Account of the Pennsylvania Hospital of Philadelphia from 1751–1938*. It was Packard's idea that a contemporary collection of medical literature for residents and interns was begun, and in 1950, the Packard Reading Room was established.

In 1974 and 1976, the Historic Library was awarded grants from the National Library of Medicine to inventory and catalog the collection for purposes of making it more

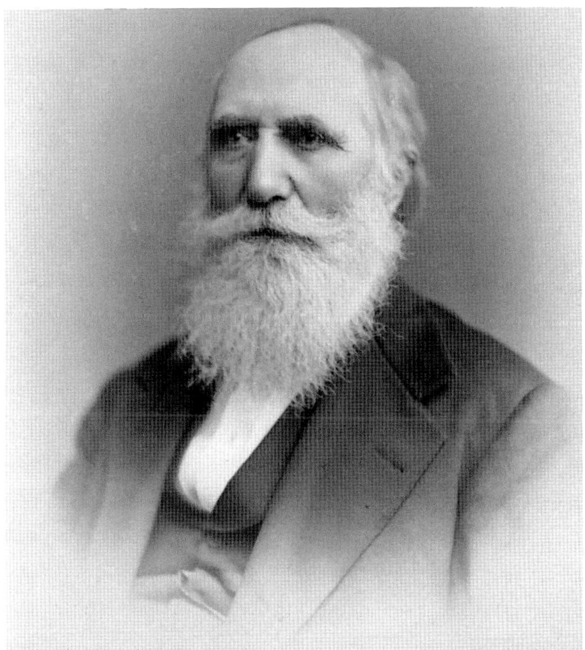

William Gunn Malin, clerk and later librarian, was the primarily influence on the growth of the library. Malin purchased subscriptions to important medical journals and prepared a comprehensive catalog of the library (1829). *Courtesy of the Pennsylvania Hospital, Philadelphia, PAH Image Collection.*

available for scholarly research. Today, the collection extends beyond the medical library. Archive materials, paintings, photographs and other memorabilia are catalogued and used regularly for research and educational exhibits. The archives include the board of manager minutes, admission and discharge records, administrative and financial records, personal correspondence of physicians and superintendents and records of other charitable organizations that were absorbed by the hospital. The memorabilia collection includes hundreds of diverse medical artifacts, including surgical kits and World War I scrapbooks from hospital nurses. The photograph collection features Dr. Thomas Kirkbride's Magic Lantern slide collection.

The Historic Library has the richest resource in early medicine of any hospital in the United States. The hospital also has one of the most comprehensive collections of nursing literature in the area. Additionally, the library is a major contributor to the National Network of Libraries of Medicine, a network exchange of healthcare information for medicine, nursing and other disciplines. Malin's tradition of professionalization continues; the contemporary library participates in union lists and surveys, and collects literature in hospital management and mental healthcare for present-day hospital staffers. It remains a repository for historic books and journal collections, with works dating from 1483 and an image archive numbering twenty-two thousand.[70]

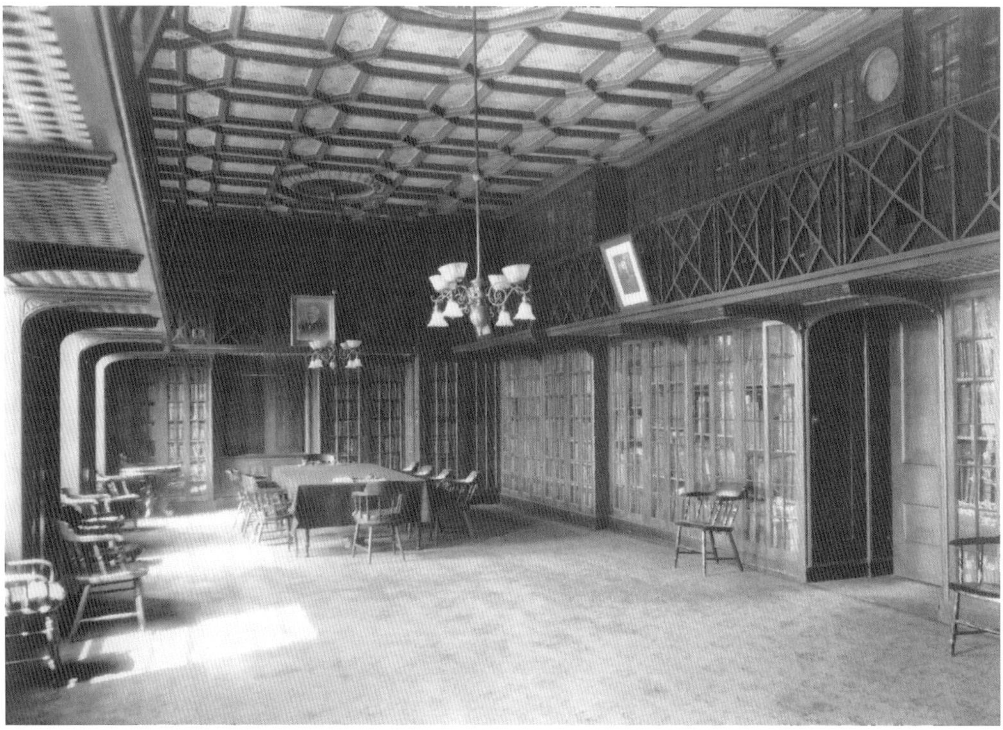

An early twentieth-century image of the Historic Library. *Courtesy of the Pennsylvania Hospital, Philadelphia, PAH Image Collection 679f.*

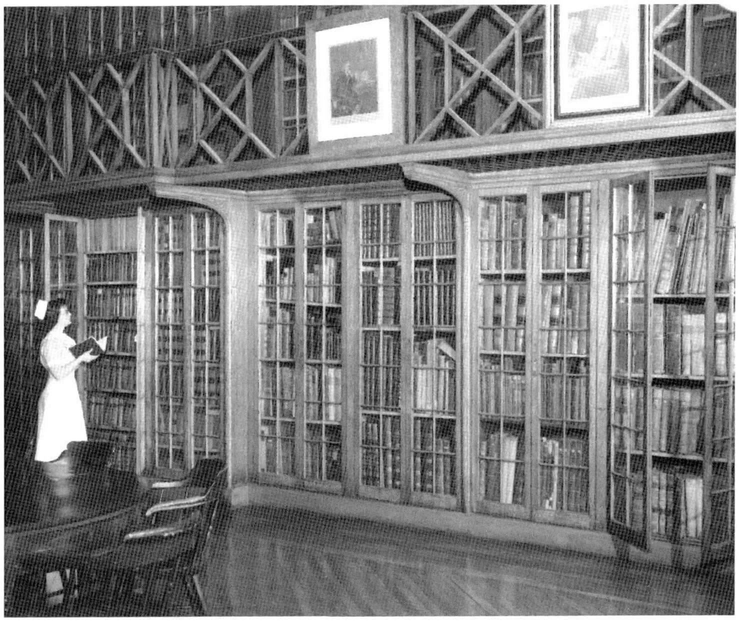

A 1957 image of a nurse reading a book in the Historic Library. Today, patrons of the Historic Library are asked to make an appointment to view material. The curator–lead archivist handles all material for patrons. *Courtesy of the Pennsylvania Hospital, Philadelphia, PAH Image Collection 681.*

THE BOARD OF MANAGERS

From Benjamin Franklin onward, Pennsylvania Hospital's board of managers was remarkable for its members—civic leaders and accomplished citizens who shared a love for and sense of responsibility about the hospital. Among its notable members was Joshua Crosby, the first president of the board, a wealthy merchant who was noted for his "humane, benevolent disposition" and his charitable nature. He laid the cornerstone of the hospital in 1755. Thomas Mifflin, who was elected to the board in 1771, was a Quaker and statesman who represented Pennsylvania in the Second Continental Congress and at the Constitutional Convention. Mifflin also served in the Continental army during the Revolutionary War and was named "President of Pennsylvania" in 1777—an office analogous to the modern position of governor.

Samuel Coates, first elected in 1785, served on the board for forty-one years. He gave up on most of his outside activities to devote himself to the running of the hospital and was known for his strong personality and work ethic. Coates was a businessman and, appropriately enough, was, in 1786, named to serve on a committee to report "on a plan of economy and on the cause of the great expense of this house." Coates was a director of the original Bank of the United States. A Quaker, Coates was particularly interested in the insane; he kept a memorandum book in which he wrote notes about cases of insane patients that were especially compelling. His good friend was Dr. Benjamin Rush, a pioneer in the field of psychiatry. But an incident early in Coates's life also piqued his interest: When he was six weeks old, a maidservant who had shown some signs of "derangement" kidnapped him. He was eventually rescued, but not before the maidservant tried to throw him out of a second-story window.[71]

Roberts Vaux, elected in 1823, was one of the originators of the public school system in Pennsylvania and the first president of the school board of Philadelphia. Vaux was a judge of the Court of Common Pleas in Philadelphia, an abolitionist and one of the founders of the Philadelphia Saving Fund Society, an asylum and school for the blind, and other benevolent institutions in the city.

Morris Cheston Sr., elected in 1942, was a member of the board for thirty-five years, and under his chairmanship, the hospital underwent a period of growth and prosperity. Cheston, an attorney, also sat on many local boards, including SmithKline Beecham and the Provident National Bank. Members of prominent Philadelphia families, including the Biddles, the Wistars and the Strawbridges, have served on the board as well.

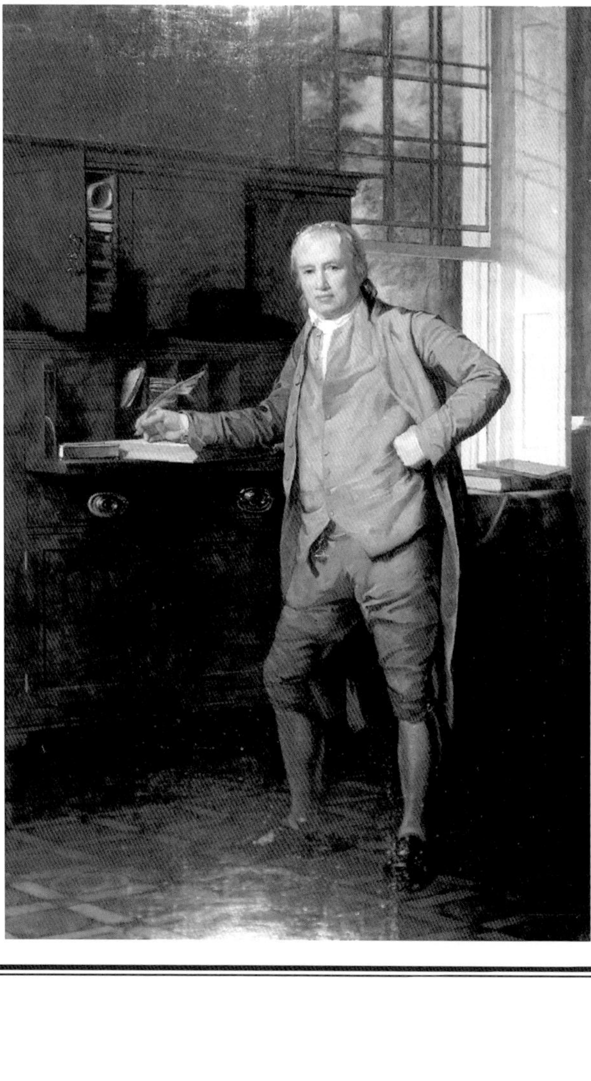

A Thomas Sully portrait of Samuel Coates, manager of the Pennsylvania Hospital. *Courtesy of the Pennsylvania Hospital, Philadelphia, PAH Image Collection 1699a.*

THE GROWING HOSPITAL, 1800–1951

THE LYING-IN WARD

By 1800, the Pennsylvania Hospital was one of only two hospitals in the country, if the term is defined as an institution dedicated exclusively to inpatient care. The other was New York Hospital, which was founded in 1771 but did not begin to receive patients until the 1790s.[72] Pennsylvania Hospital marked a milestone in 1803, when its lying-in, or maternity ward, was opened on the second floor, East Wing, of the Pine Building. The Pennsylvania Assembly had authorized the hospital to establish such a department in 1793, but there was some dissention among the managers. Some thought it improper for a pregnant woman to be attended by a male; others felt that the hospital starting such a ward would be a tacit stamp of approval for poor, unwed mothers to turn to vice and immorality.

Then there was the problem of limited finances. The proposal was taken back up again in late 1802, and the lying-in ward was begun in 1803. Dr. Thomas Chalkey James was named first physician to the Lying-in Department, and obstetrics was the first named specialty at the hospital. The Lying-in Department operated until 1854, when widespread outbreaks of puerperal fever caused it to close.[73] Affiliations with other lying-in units would be established in the late nineteenth century, and much later, in 1960, the hospital would affiliate with the Preston Retreat.

THE DREADED CIRCULAR ROOM

In 1804, the managers laid out a plan for the systematic maintenance of medical histories. They ordered a record book containing notes about each case "which shall

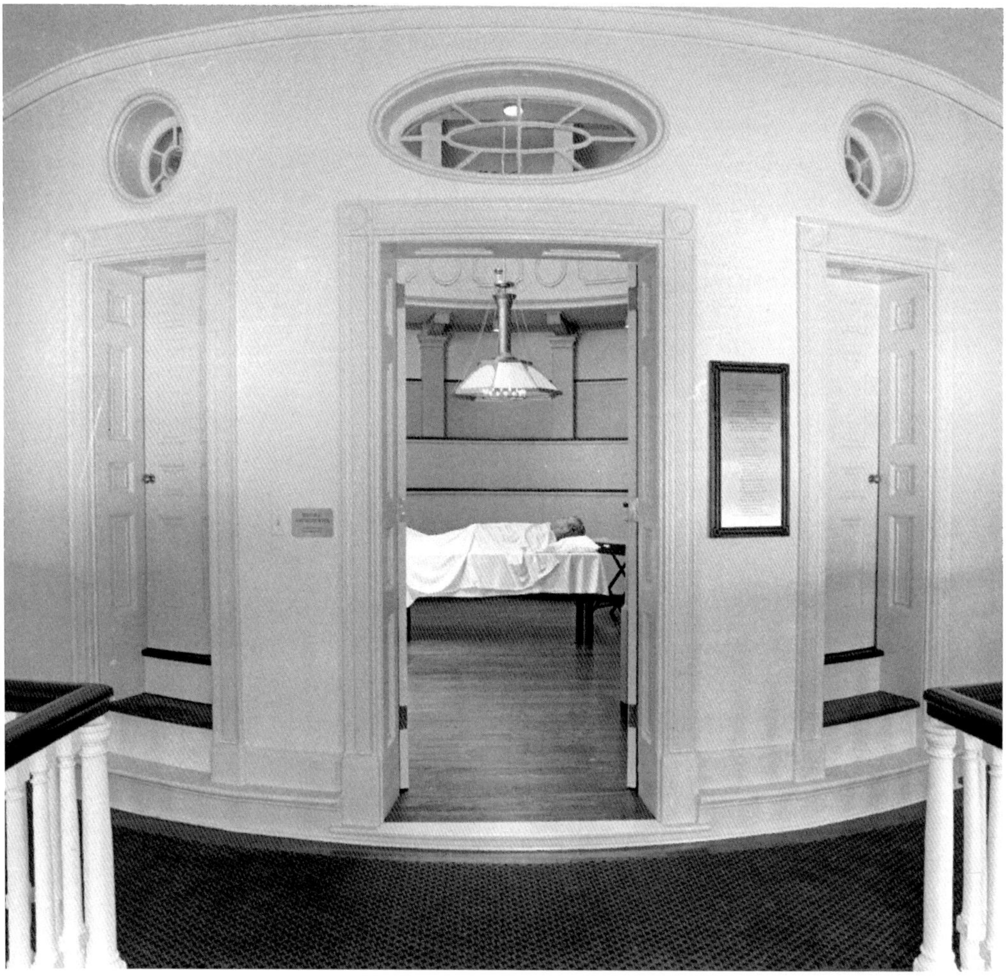

A promotional picture of the exterior of the surgical amphitheatre after restoration in 1977. *Courtesy of the Pennsylvania Hospital, Philadelphia, PAH Image Collection.*

be the property of the Contributors (not to be lent out) but, laid before the managers at every one of their monthly meetings."[74]

The hospital achieved another milestone in 1804, when the surgical amphitheatre was completed in the center of the Pine Building. It was the first such room of its kind in the United States. There were no provisions for surgery in the oldest wing, the East Wing; all available space was used for staff or housing patients. The large, third-floor, circular amphitheatre was the final portion of the center section to open. Instead of a dome to top the building, it was decided that a skylight for the amphitheatre would be a better choice. Thirty feet high and twenty-eight feet in diameter, the amphitheatre contained an upper gallery with rows of wooden benches for students and observers, who paid one guinea for admittance to watch surgeons amputate limbs, remove tumors or set broken bones. The benches overflowed when a curious operation or a popular lecture was on tap. Since the amphitheatre was lit only by natural light, operations were scheduled

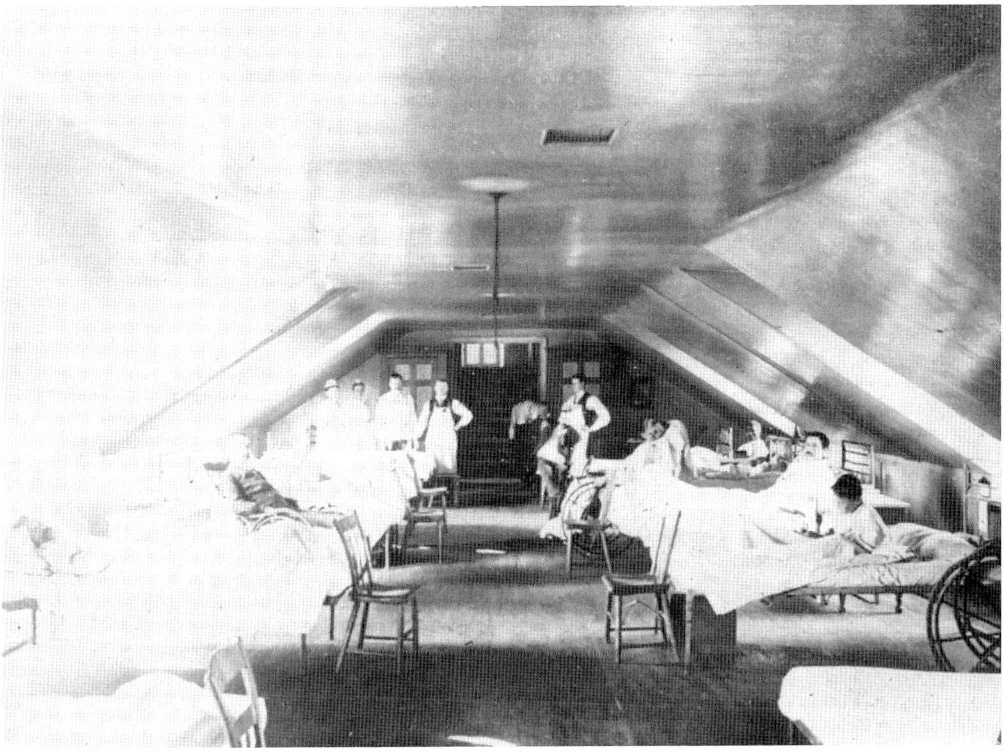

An 1894 image of the upper surgical ward (East Wing). This area is used as the archives today. *Courtesy of the Pennsylvania Hospital, Philadelphia, PAH Image Collection.*

for midday, between 11:00 a.m. and 2:00 p.m., typically during clear weather. (There was never enough light in the room for minute work, such as was required during eye operations, so those were conducted in another room.)[75]

Procedures were performed in an unsterile atmosphere, since sterile conditions were not widely used until about 1900—neither surgeon's hands nor their instruments received more than a rudimentary cleaning, and in those days, before the acceptance of Joseph Lister's theory that germs caused infection, surgeons typically washed up after surgery. Clinical aids such as the stethoscope were not yet available. And until anesthesia came to the hospital in about 1840, patients were either given opium or liquor, or "administered them a sharp tap on the head with a mallet enough to render the patient unconscious and hopefully not dead."[76] Patients were typically tied down to the operating table and then kept from moving by burly attendants; the mark of a good surgeon in those days was a man's quickness with his knife. Typically, patients were so weakened from the blood loss of surgery that they would not return to the wards below but to the "apartment" —the first recovery room in the country, adjoining the surgery, where they might regain their strength. There is little doubt why the room was known as the "Dreaded Circular Room."[77]

It was in this room that Dr. Philip Syng Physick made his mark. A physician at Pennsylvania Hospital since 1794, he excelled at surgery and is known today as the

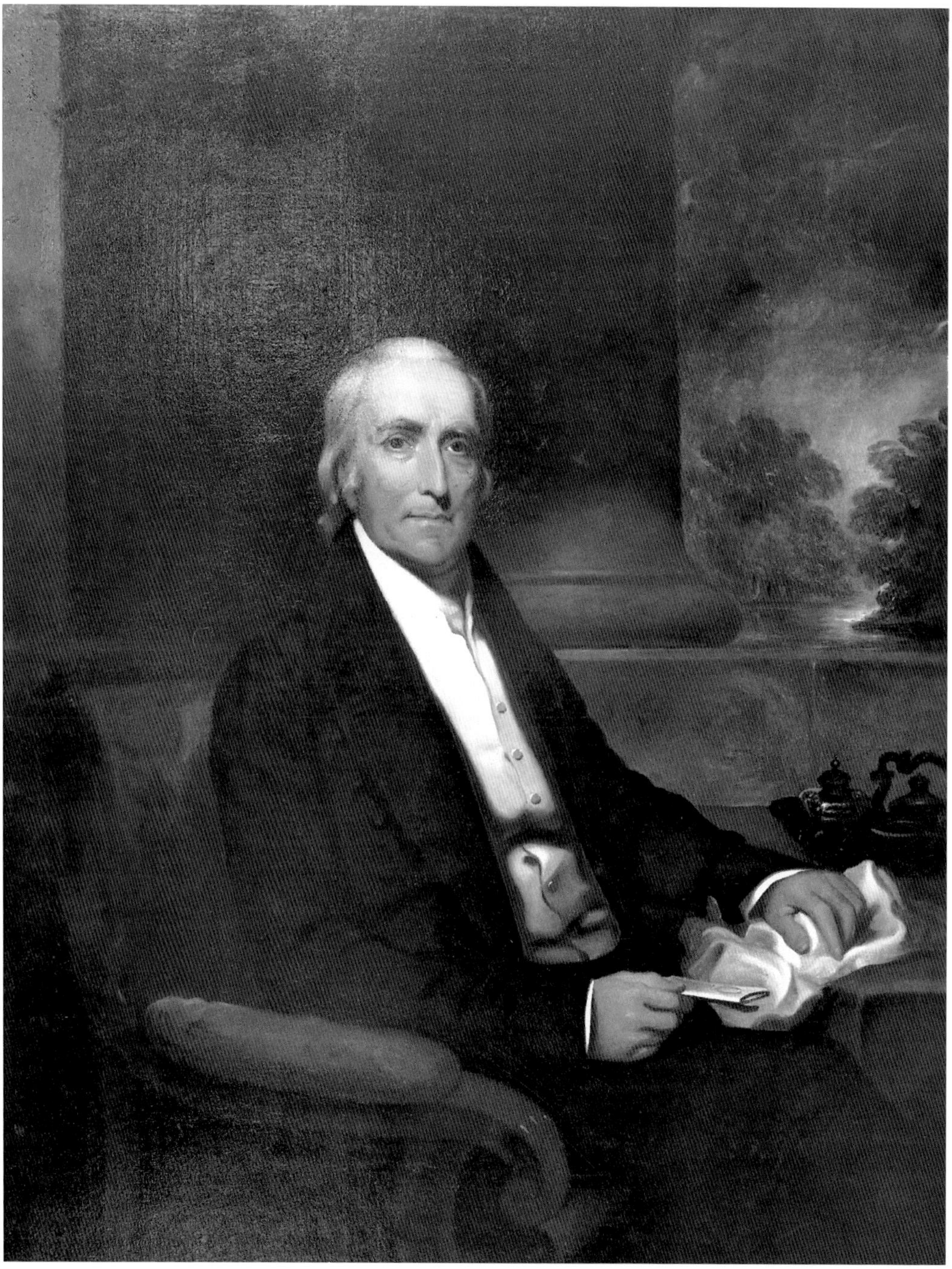

A portrait of Dr. Philip Syng Physick, known as the "Father of American Surgery." The seven-pound tumor Dr. Physick removed from a patient in 1805 is still on view in the Pine Building. *Courtesy of the Pennsylvania Hospital, Philadelphia, PAH Image Collection 1706.*

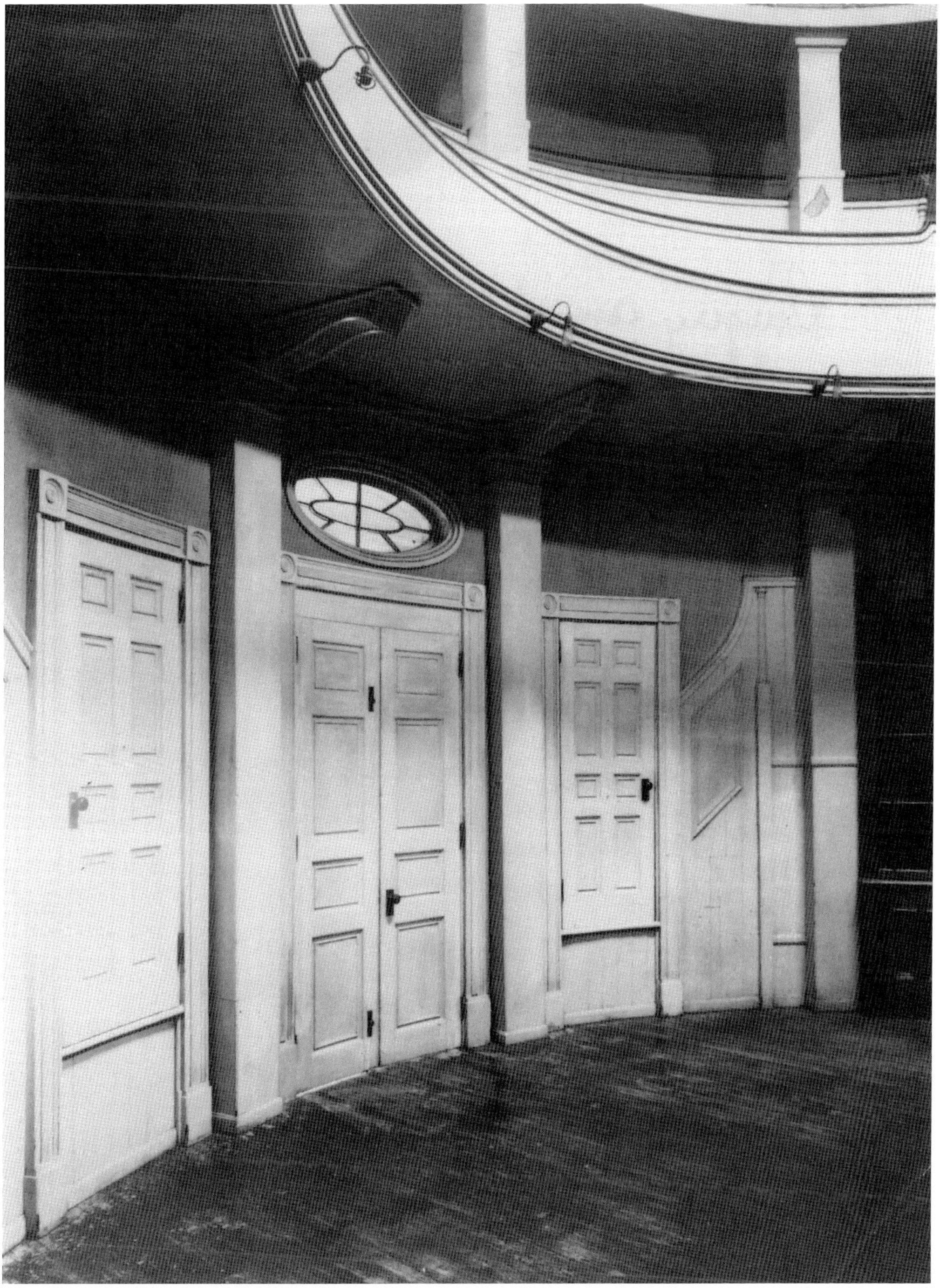

The Historic Amphitheatre prior to restoration work. *Courtesy of the Pennsylvania Hospital, Philadelphia, PAH Image Collection.*

"father of American Surgery." As a surgeon, he is described as "having a correct, sharp and discriminating eye; a hand delicate in touch, dexterous in movement and of unswerving firmness; a perfect composure and self-possession which rose in tone and deepened in steadiness with the complication of the case at hand."[78] Physick was renowned for his prowess in operations on the eye, but he is perhaps best known for performing a successful lithotomy on Chief Justice John Marshall in 1831. The outcome of the operation so pleased Marshall that he presented Physick with a silver wine cooler. Physick was also known for removing a seven-pound tumor from a man's face and for inventing the tonsil guillotine, an instrument used to remove tonsils.[79]

The surgical amphitheatre helped change the face of clinical medical education—with its advent, students could see patients in front of them in the lecture room. Dr. Benjamin Coates began the practice of demonstrating with patients in 1834, a policy that followed closely Dr. Thomas Bond's bedside clinical teaching, which had happened at Pennsylvania Hospital since its first days. The opening of the amphitheatre, however, marked the beginning of surgery as a recognized discipline, and the amphitheatre filled a long-held desire by the University of Pennsylvania's faculty for a room in which a large class could receive formal lectures and observe surgeries. Some called Philadelphia

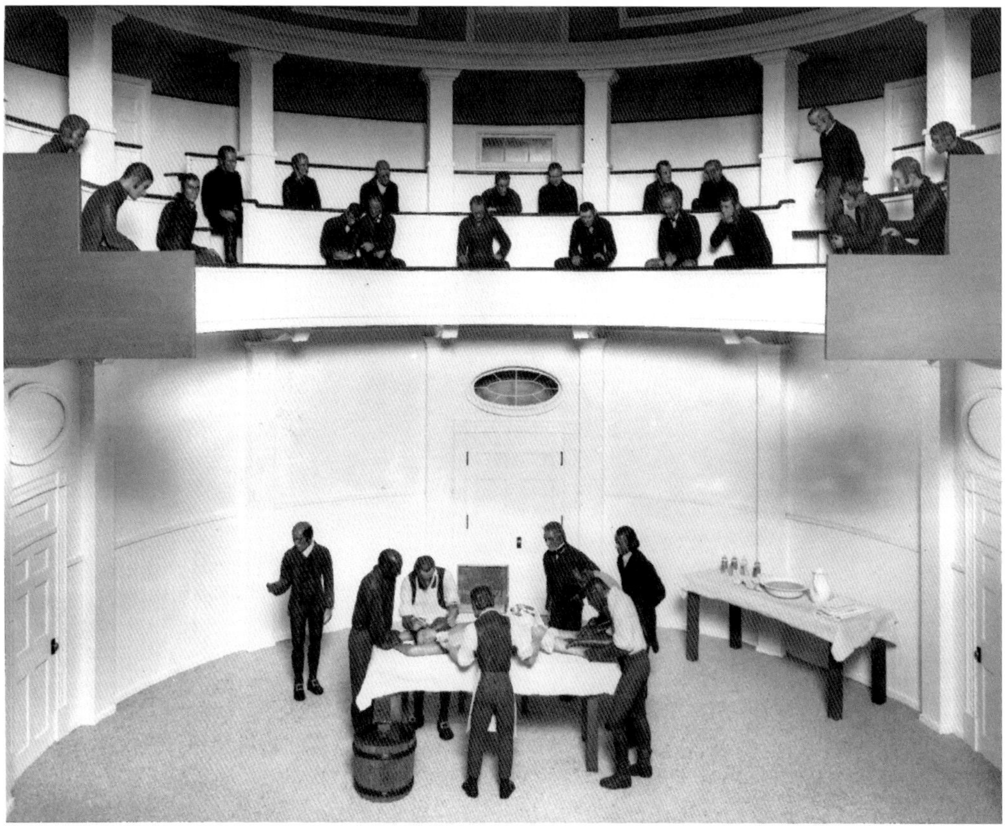

A diorama (1964) of the Historic Amphitheatre at the Smithsonian. *Courtesy of the Pennsylvania Hospital, Philadelphia, PAH Image Collection 565.*

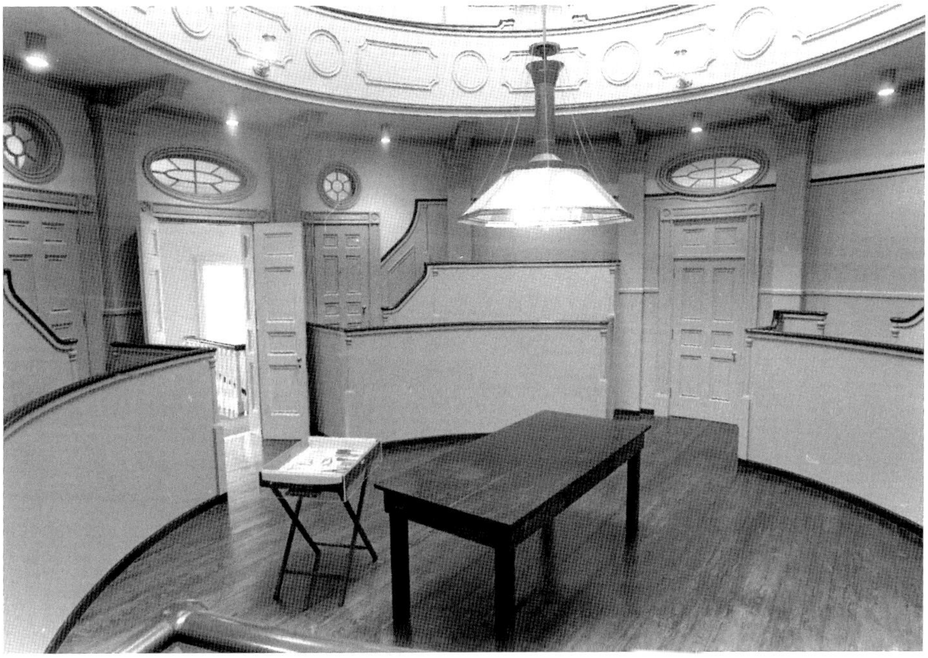

The Historic Amphitheatre after renovation. *Courtesy of the Pennsylvania Hospital, Philadelphia, PAH Image Collection 565.1.*

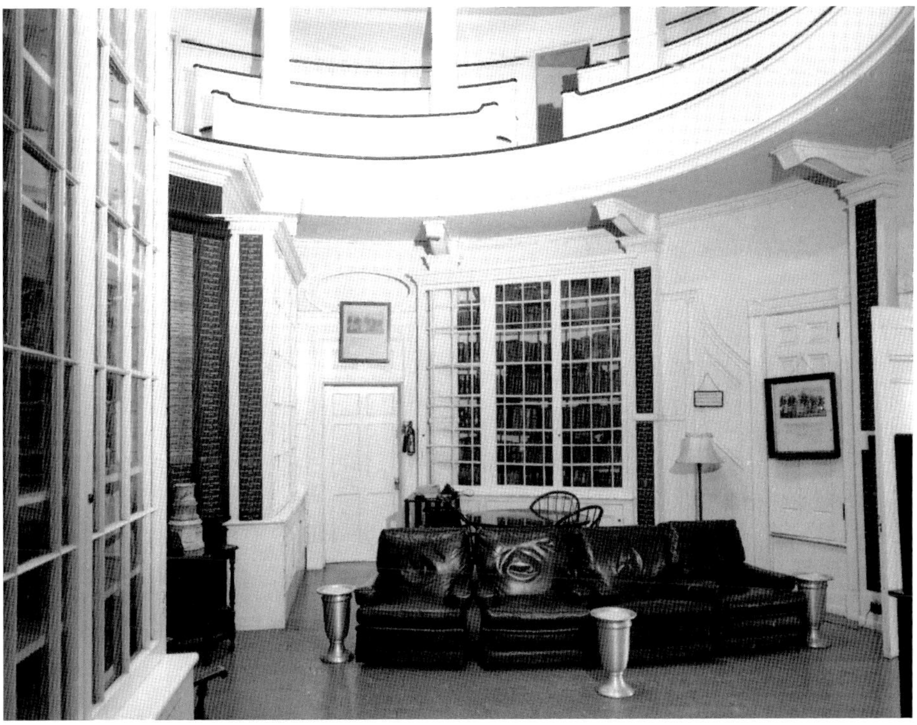

In the mid-twentieth century, the Historic Amphitheatre was used as a lounge for residents. This image was taken in 1960. Notice the curve of the walls and the balcony at the top of the image. *Courtesy of the Pennsylvania Hospital, Philadelphia, PAH Image Collection 564.*

"the Athens of America" because it attracted students seeking medical education and clinical instruction not available anywhere else in the country. The amphitheatre ceased hosting surgeries in 1868, when another, larger amphitheatre opened in another part of the hospital. The room has been a dining room for nurses and patients, a lounge for the house staff and, since 1976, when funds were raised to renovate the space, it has appeared as it did in the nineteenth century. Visitors are welcome in the grand space.[80]

WAR OF 1812

During the War of 1812, Pennsylvania Hospital was again called upon by military authorities for aid. An April 1814 letter from Alexander Walker Jr., agent for British prisoners, stated that he "had paid for the Board of Wounded Prisoners Sent to the Hospital." Walker wanted to know whether the hospital was supported chiefly by private contributions, not by federal money.[81] A number of British prisoners and American sailors were treated at the hospital in 1814.

BOARD OF FEMALE ASSISTANTS

In 1824, the hospital established the "Board of Female Assistants for the Internal Management of the Hospital," a group comprising Amy Coates, Mary Cope, Catharine W. Morris and Beulah Sansom and charged with visiting patients and reporting back suggestions for improvement "as they may judge salutary, useful or needful." The hospital seemed to look favorably upon the advice of that board. But in 1827, a clash between the female board and the board of managers occurred. The ladies "expressed their disapproval of retaining a certain employee in the hospital in any capacity whatsoever." It seems that the employee was operating room nurse Sarah Malin, though the reason she fell out of favor was not recorded.

The managers refused to accept the women's judgment, however, and the female board resigned in a body, stating that "under the existing circumstances we can render you no acceptable or efficient aid."[82] The managers then declared the female board abolished.[83] Another forty years passed before the women's committee, a precursor to the women's auxiliary and made up of a group of "Christian women," was formed. That group was organized to aid the mental, moral and spiritual needs of patients at the hospital, though they were not to make any changes themselves, instead bringing suggestions to the board of managers.[84]

CONDITIONS IN THE EARLY NINETEENTH CENTURY

Early in the nineteenth century, Pennsylvania Hospital found itself caught between the need to specialize and expand its physical facilities and the unwillingness of the government to support such changes. It was up to the board of managers to find a way out. A 1796 state grant marked the end of direct public assistance to the hospital until the twentieth century. Besides the lack of support, the city, county and federal government all attempted to make the hospital pay taxes.

In 1808, the city and county of Philadelphia assessed the hospital for the first time. The board refused to pay, and the tax collector seized some of the hospital's cows and hay. Managers appealed to state legislators, who did not intervene. In 1814, federal lawmakers readied a bill to place a federal tax on all property taxed by county governments. Finally, in 1816, after the hospital had paid a year's worth of taxes, a public petition convinced state legislators to grant the hospital a tax exemption. The hospital relied on private donations to make up for the lack of government aid. The largest individual benefactor was Stephen Girard, a merchant and banker whose first wife was an insane patient at the hospital. Between 1786 and 1816, Girard gave more than $4,000, and in 1832, he left the hospital $29,250 in his will.

The city's population boom meant that the managers could no longer know the vast majority of applicants for admission. Admissions were likely less selective as a result, but managers still rejected patients who were contagious or chronically ill. (Lepers, however, were admitted.)[85] And though they could not know each patient personally, the managers still remained vigilant. In 1817, when an oversight led to an unmarried female in the Lying-in Department, the board resolved that in the future "no person be admitted to the benefit of that department unless satisfactory evidence be produced of her living in lawful wedlock, and that she did so at the period of her becoming pregnant."

Even physicians did not have final say over who was admitted. When a friend asked Dr. Benjamin Rush for help with an admission, Dr. Rush promised only that he would plead the patient's case.[86] Often, a patient's social network determined whether he was worthy of admission or bound for the almshouse. Membership in a certain church, service to a particular family or pleasing personal characteristics could help a patient's chances of admission. In 1853, a prominent Philadelphian recommended a Mrs. Milne for admission to the hospital. She was the wife of a talented but alcoholic shoemaker. "I have known Mrs. Milne since four or five years: and she is well known to Mrs. Jackson, my sister Mrs. Henry, to Mrs. [Buckley], and to many other ladies. I believe we can all testify that she is deserving, industrious, well-behaved and respectable."[87]

At the turn of the century, paying patients made up 65 percent of the hospital's patient roster, but in 1840, by which time the hospital's finances had improved, the figure was 40 percent. Patients were segregated, with venereal patients occupying an outbuilding. African Americans were also segregated during this time. Those who did not reside in Pennsylvania were charged one dollar per week more than Pennsylvania residents. The sick poor could be admitted one of three ways: If empty beds were available, a patient could meet the criteria for nonpaying patients. (This was made easier in 1809, when the burial and clothing deposit was abolished.) They could also be admitted as paying patients under the sponsorship of an agency. The third way was to be sponsored by a private patron. Patients were still accommodated in open wards of up to twenty-five beds, with no curtains between beds.[88]

Civil War

When the Civil War began in 1861, Pennsylvania Hospital was again called upon to treat the wounded. In fact, the first casualty it received came not from a battle but from an act of secessionist mob violence in Baltimore. Private George Leisenring died at Pennsylvania Hospital four days after sustaining injuries in a Baltimore train station. The mob had seized upon a Philadelphia contingent of Northern recruits, and Leisenring became the first casualty.[89]

At the annual managers' meeting in 1861, the board of managers made a statement that read in part:

> *At the present time, when our country is threatened with the terrible scourge, war, it behooves us to endeavor to be prepared by every means in our power, to relieve those who may be sufferers from the inseparable ills which must follow in its train, and that not one applicant should be allowed to leave our gate while there is room to accommodate, because the funds adequate to relieve are wanted.*

A few months later, the managers said they could take 60 soldier patients at once and would soon be ready for 80 additional. They also offered authorities room to build a temporary hospital, if it was necessary. The hospital admitted 124 wounded or sick soldiers between July 7 and October 13, 1862, many of whom were specialized surgical cases, given Pennsylvania Hospital's excellent reputation for surgery.[90]

As it had during the Revolutionary War, the hospital suffered economically during and after the Civil War. Across the board, charitable institutions were not properly funded, financially or supply-wise. The Department of the Insane received no reimbursement for the large number of Southern patients it housed.[91]

Medical Advances

Medical advances continued apace during this time. The first operation deliberately removing a diseased appendix was performed at the hospital in 1887 by Dr. Thomas

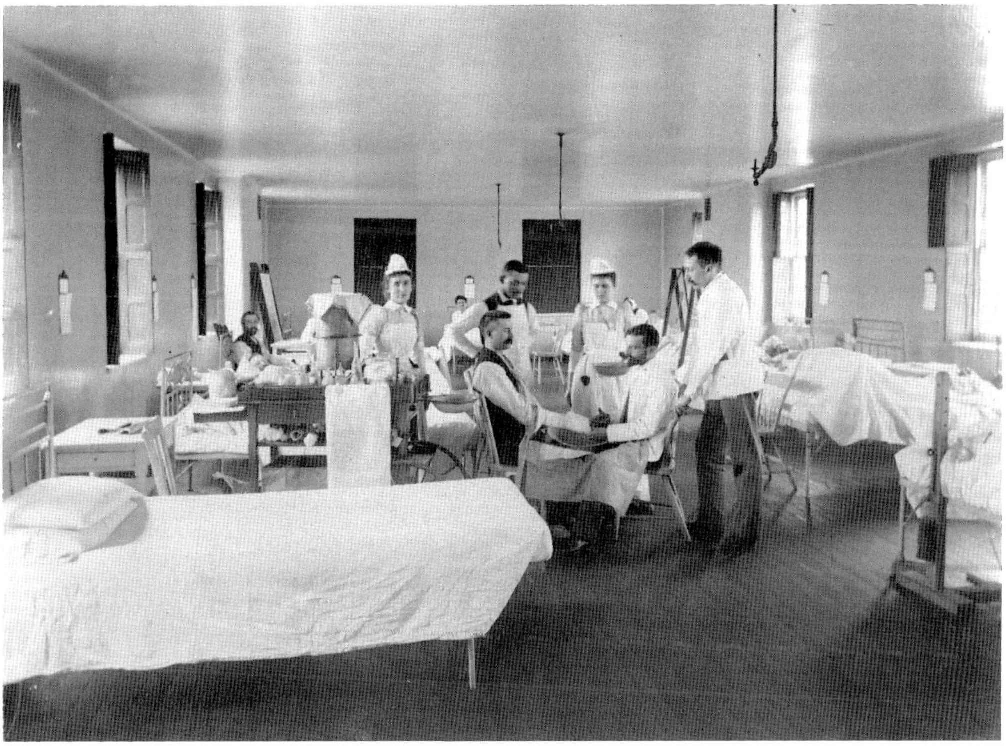

An 1893 image of the Emergency Ward. *Courtesy of the Pennsylvania Hospital, Philadelphia, PAH Image Collection 715.*

Morton. In 1911, Dr. R.G. LeConte performed the first American thoracoplasty in the case of tuberculosis of the lungs—a procedure removing some of the ribs to produce a collapse of the diseased lung in order to circumscribe the disease.[92]

The 1880s to the 1920s saw a transformation in the American hospital, and Pennsylvania Hospital was no exception. Hospitals were originally facilities for the long-term care of the chronically ill, but during this time, they became scientific facilities for acute intervention. The number of hospitals increased, and patients were increasingly middle class and paying. Medicine advanced, too. Diagnostic laboratories gave doctors the ability to identify with confidence specific microbial disease. Advances in anesthesiology and asepsis, and new medical technology like the X-ray and the electrocardiogram, allowed physicians to confidently monitor its function.

In 1897, two years after Wilhelm Roentgen's description of the X-ray amazed the Western world, the hospital purchased its first X-ray machine. It was a symbol of advanced scientific medicine. The machine, which was described in medical literature as being useful for diagnosing abnormal bone conditions, was slow to make an impact on patient care—at first, it was merely a curiosity. The chief resident was charged with operating the machine, among his many other tasks. But by 1912, one physician on staff was given the job of operating the X-ray machine. An X-ray department was established, and a radiographer in charge was engaged. By 1917, the X-ray had become

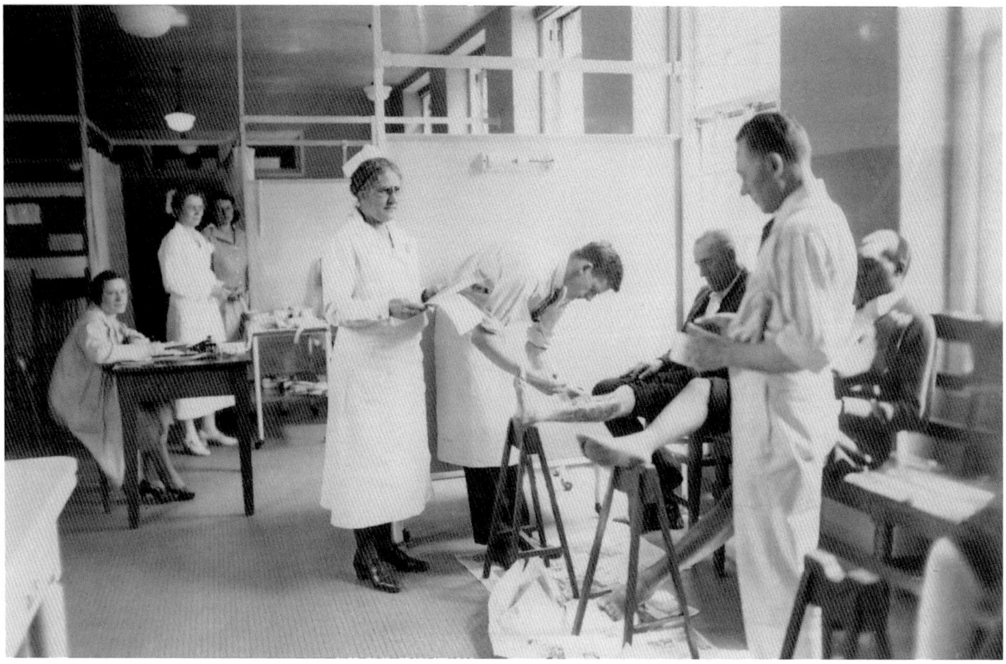

Tending to patients, 1936. *Courtesy of the Pennsylvania Hospital, Philadelphia, PAH Image Collection.*

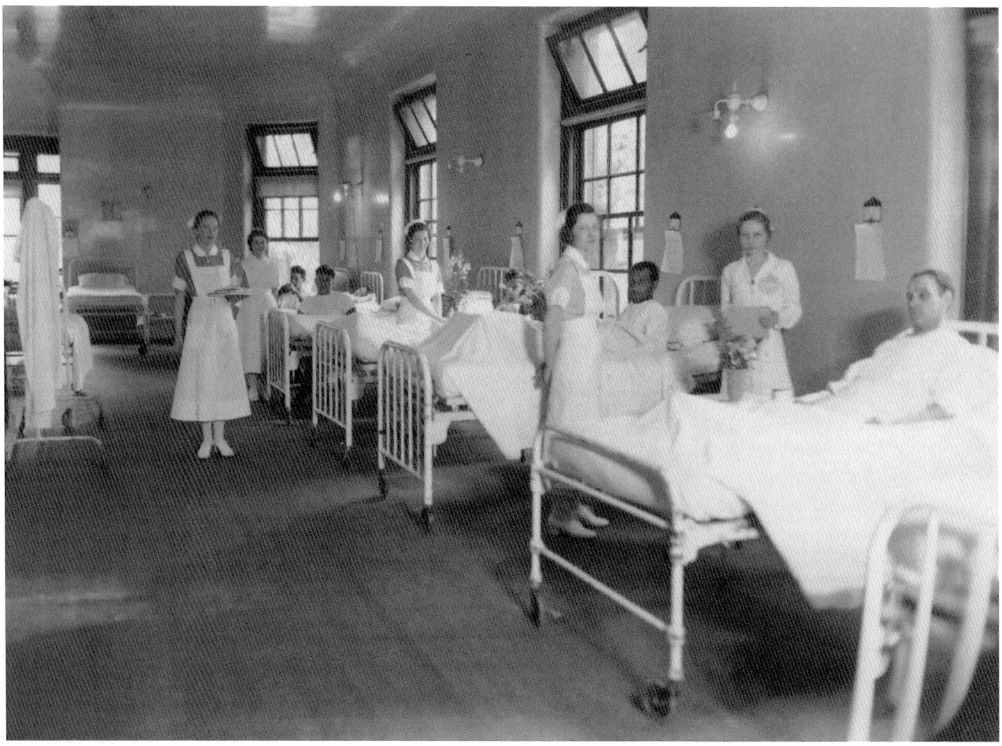

Nurses tending to patients, 1936. *Courtesy of the Pennsylvania Hospital, Philadelphia, PAH Image Collection.*

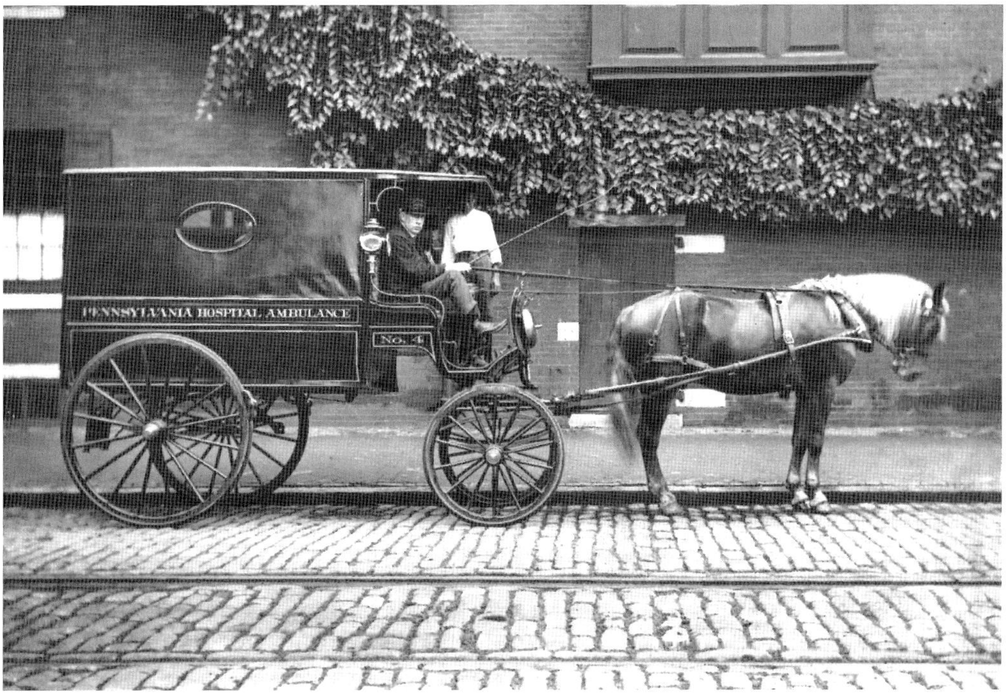

Horse-drawn ambulance #4 by the streetcar tracks on Eighth Street. *Courtesy of the Pennsylvania Hospital, Philadelphia, PAH Image Collection 2620.1.*

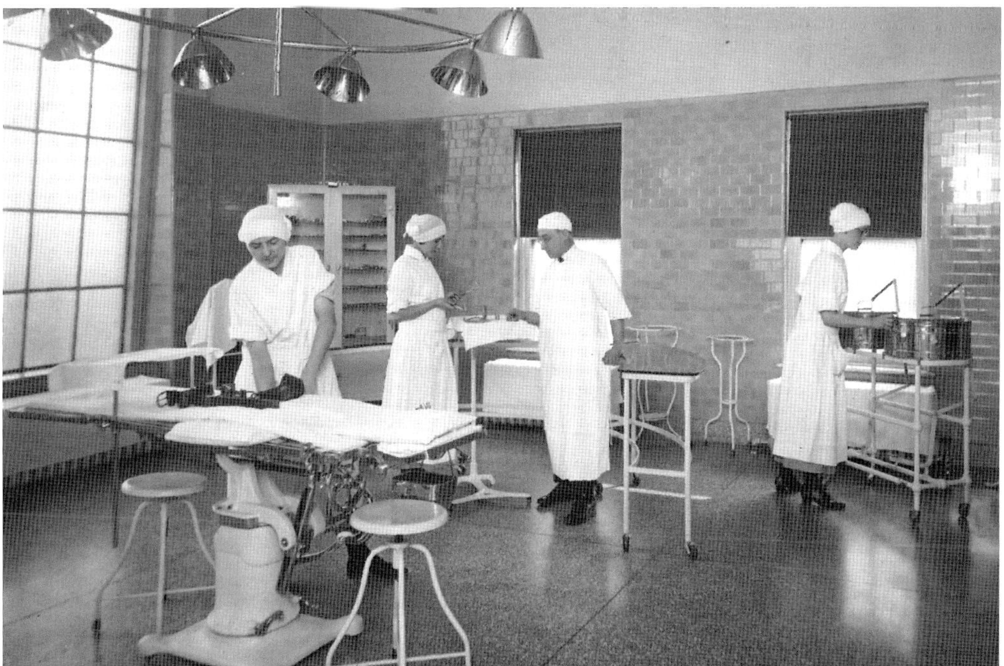

An example of an operating room from the 1920s. *Courtesy of the Pennsylvania Hospital, Philadelphia, PAH Image Collection.*

a routine diagnostic test for patients with kidney stones or limb fractures. World War I increased the X-ray's importance, with more use by Pennsylvania Hospital doctors and nurses overseas and more technological advances in the machine itself, including the development of a portable X-ray machine.

Similarly, the development of an electrocardiogram, or ECG, machine to record the electrical action of the human heart brought advances to the hospital. The first ECG machine was purchased in 1921, and by the latter part of that decade, it was well on its way to becoming a routine part of patient care. The ECG department expanded rapidly, a sign that technology was now quicker to catch on than in the days when the X-ray machine was first purchased.

Patient records were becoming more sophisticated, too. By 1927, the results of diagnostic tests were reported on separate, standardized forms, often with graphs or pictures. Test results were now typed up and signed by a specialist. Standardization and quantification became important, and the old way of having a single intern handwrite each record was obsolete.[93]

SPANISH-AMERICAN WAR

The Spanish-American War of 1898 was brief—it lasted just eight months—but it again tested the hospital's ability to efficiently handle large numbers of patients. Hospital administrators offered to care for sick and wounded soldiers, but they were told initially that their services would not be needed. That changed quickly, however. "During the past month [July 1898] the facilities of the Hospital have been tried as never before since its capacity has increased, and we have again had an opportunity to witness the ability of the Hospital to meet emergencies," hospital superintendent Daniel Test wrote. In that month, 179 soldiers were treated; in September and October, 113 more were admitted. Most suffered from typhoid fever.[94] Some were transported on special Red Cross trains manned by Pennsylvania Hospital staff.

AYER CLINICAL LABORATORY

In 1898 a $50,000 bequest from Josephine Mellon Ayer made possible the opening of the Ayer Clinical Laboratory. The clinical laboratory became important to medicine by 1900, when technology advanced to the point where examining some part of the living patient—excretions, blood or secretions—helped physicians reach a diagnosis or provide better treatment. In 1870, the average physician knew little chemistry and could

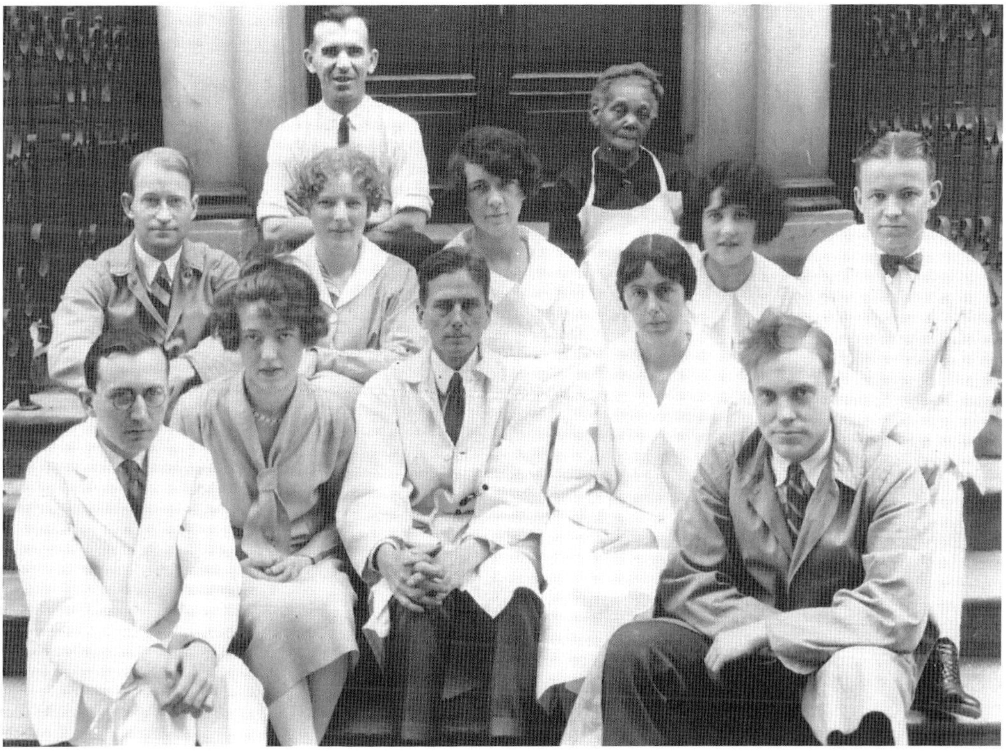

Staff of the Ayer Laboratory, 1926. *Courtesy of the Pennsylvania Hospital, Philadelphia, PAH Image Collection.*

probably not use a microscope. By 1900, microscopes were widely used, as their value became more recognized over the years and hospitals invested money in equipment and personnel. Clinical laboratories such as Ayer advanced medicine in that they contributed precise information about patients. They also advanced the understanding of disease as it manifests in living patients.[95]

THE HOSPITAL DURING WORLD WAR I

Out of the Geneva Convention of 1863 and a strong desire to better organize American hospitals came the American Red Cross, an organization that would have an impact on Pennsylvania Hospital and its war efforts. The suffering of the sick and wounded in the Civil and Spanish-American Wars demonstrated the need for better hospital preparation, and as "the Great War" played on the world stage beginning in 1914, it was clear that hospitals would have to play a crucial role in the war effort.

Pennsylvania Hospital was at the forefront of preparation for America's entry into World War I as one of the first hospital service units organized under the auspices of the American Red Cross.[96] In 1916, Base Hospital No. 10 was organized with the blessing of the board of managers and $25,000 worth of equipment from the Pennsylvania Committee for National Preparedness. When war was declared on April 6, 1917, the unit was quickly readied. Margaret A. Dunlop, director of nurses at Pennsylvania Hospital, had just five days to ready a cadre of nurses from her graduates and a group of nurses from other Philadelphia hospitals. In charge of doctors and enlisted men was Dr. Richard H. Harte; both Dunlop and Dr. Harte had wartime experience, having served at the American Ambulance Hospital at Neuilly, France. Their unit was ready within a few days, and on May 16, it received orders. Two days later, it was on the way to France.

The unit arrived at Le Treport and took over British General Hospital No. 16, a well-equipped hospital with a two-thousand-bed capacity. Since the unit itself could only handle five hundred beds, officers cabled for reinforcements, and it remained at Le Treport until February 1919, when it returned to the United States. In all, the unit cared for more than forty-six thousand sick and wounded patients, mostly British Expeditionary Forces and three thousand Americans. Mortality was quite low, with just 538 deaths. Six members of the unit—Kenneth Hay, Helen Fairchild, Paul Acosta, James Allen, Frank Dochney and John Wesley Thomas—died in service to their country.[97]

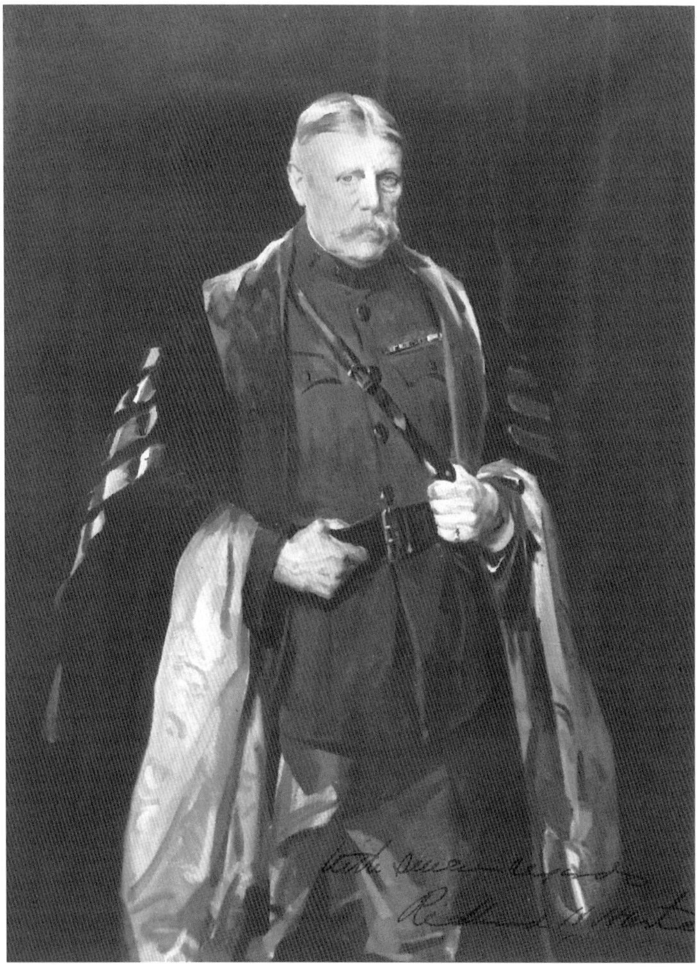

A portrait of Dr. Richard H. Harte by Leopold Seffert. This portrait was awarded the R. Proctor Prize in the National Academy of Design's New York show. *Courtesy of the Pennsylvania Hospital, Philadelphia, PAH School of Nursing Collection MG 3.13 ff57.*

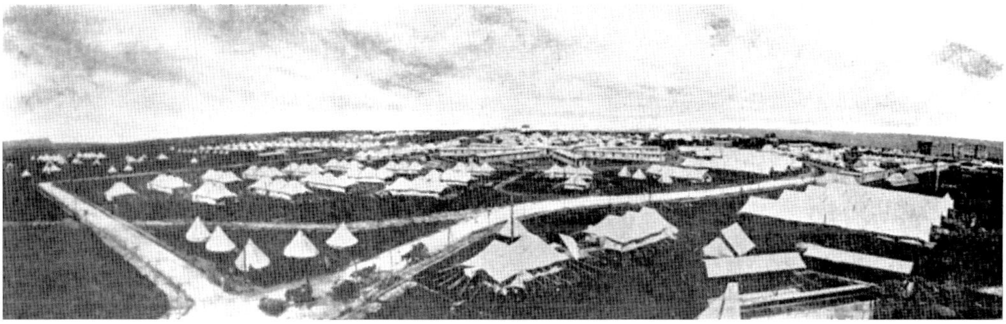

A panoramic view of the Base 10 Hospital in Le Treport, France, during World War I. *Courtesy of the Pennsylvania Hospital, Philadelphia, PAH School of Nursing Collection MG3.11 ff161, Anna Dean Murphy Collection, not dated.*

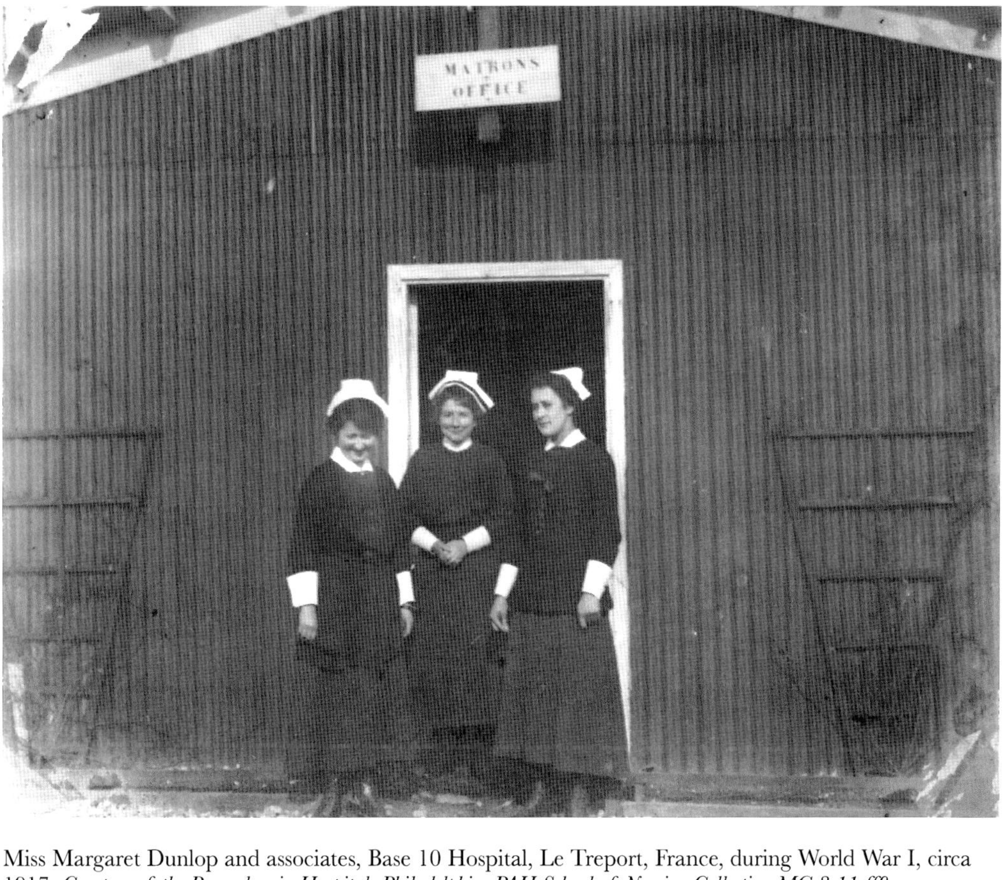

Miss Margaret Dunlop and associates, Base 10 Hospital, Le Treport, France, during World War I, circa 1917. *Courtesy of the Pennsylvania Hospital, Philadelphia; PAH School of Nursing Collection MG 3.11 ff8.*

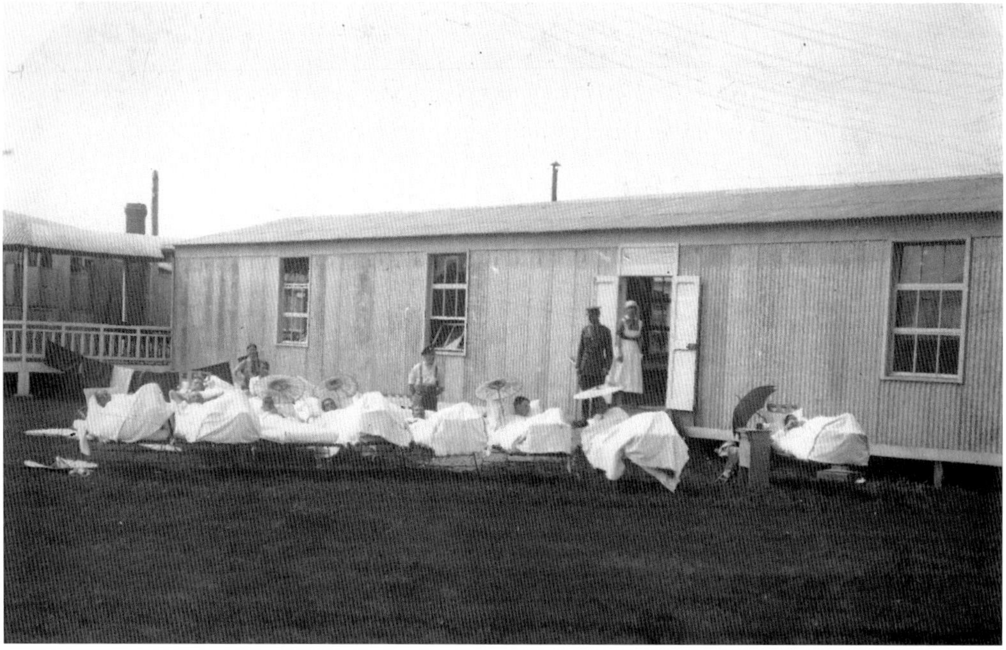

Patients resting outside Base 10 Hospital, Le Treport, France, during World War I. *Courtesy of the Pennsylvania Hospital, Philadelphia; PAH Image Collection 1672.*

At home, the hospital ran at about half strength, hampered by low staff and a large number of sick sailors in the wards. The worldwide influenza epidemic hit Pennsylvania Hospital in October 1918, striking the already depleted nursing staff with special force. Fifty-two nurses became ill and four died.[98] That fall, third-year and fourth-year medical students at the University of Pennsylvania School of Medicine were given a single lecture on influenza and told their classes had been suspended, and then they opened a makeshift hospital in the city, with third-year students serving as nurses and fourth-years as doctors. For five weeks, they worked with little supervision in the presence of alarming patient mortality. Still, their work allowed the hospital to remain open.[99]

ADVANCES IN OUTPATIENT CARE

In 1927, a new outpatient building on the south side of Spruce Street was opened. This marked the affiliation of the historic Philadelphia Dispensary—an institution opened in 1786 to serve outpatients at Fifth and Market—with Pennsylvania Hospital. Though the hospital treated its first outpatient in 1752, a patient who suffered from "a case of periodical Madness,"[100] it was not until the Philadelphia Dispensary opened that a formal outpatient department was organized at the hospital. From 1818 to 1872, there was a lapse in outpatient services at the hospital. The City of Philadelphia had established several dispensaries on its own by this time, and the hospital's services languished. But in 1872, outpatient services were resumed when the hospital established them in a building known as the "Retreat" in the northwest corner of the hospital's grounds. Outpatient services were located here until 1879, when the hospital purchased a lot on the north side of Spruce Street and erected a building there.[101] The department remained there until the affiliation with the Philadelphia Dispensary in 1927. During this time, the hospital also got back in the "baby business," reinstating obstetrics and gynecology with the new Women's Building, opened in 1929.

THE HOSPITAL DURING WORLD WAR II

Keeping its tradition of serving its country during wartime, Pennsylvania Hospital answered the call of duty during World War II. Before the country entered the war, hospital administrators received a request from the U.S. surgeon general to sponsor the Fifty-second Evacuation Hospital as part of the War Department's Protective Mobilization Plan. The board accepted the invitation, naming Dr. Charles F. Mitchell to organize the new group. He would be aided by Helen G. McClelland, RN, who organized the nursing arm of the unit. The Fifty-second began with forty-seven medical officers, fifty-two nurse officers and three hundred enlisted men. Some personnel from other Philadelphia hospitals joined the group as well. They were not the only Pennsylvania Hospital personnel to serve in the war—others left at different times to serve in every branch of the armed forces, in every theatre of the war.[102]

Two weeks after the Japanese bombed Pearl Harbor on December 7, 1941, and the United States formally entered the war, the unit was called into action. It was the first convoy to sail for the Pacific theatre. The unit arrived at a small village on the island of New Caledonia and quickly set up a makeshift hospital in huts constructed by hospital personnel with the aid of some locals. Despite obsolete equipment and a lack of vital materials, the hospital still managed to treat more than six thousand patients in just six months. Later, in the fall of 1942, a forward unit was established in Noumea. Its small staff quickly took care of over two thousand patients.

In time, medical officers from the Fifty-second were sent out to Guadalcanal to relieve staff in field hospitals there. Nurses were dispatched to the U.S. Navy Hospital ship *Solace* at various times. The unit served in many locations in the Pacific, including Woodlast Island, off New Guinea, Finschaefer and the Philippines.[103]

As with many previous wars, World War II took a steep toll on the hospital. Hospital administrator John N. Hatfield, in his 1944 annual report, wrote of an "overworked and undermanned" surgical staff and the closure of parts of some wards for several months. Still, the damage was less than it could have been—a huge volunteer corps kept the hospital going, warding off the closure of more of the hospital for longer periods of time. The United States Nurse Cadet Corps, in particular, helped the hospital during this time of scarce personnel resources. The national program provided funding for

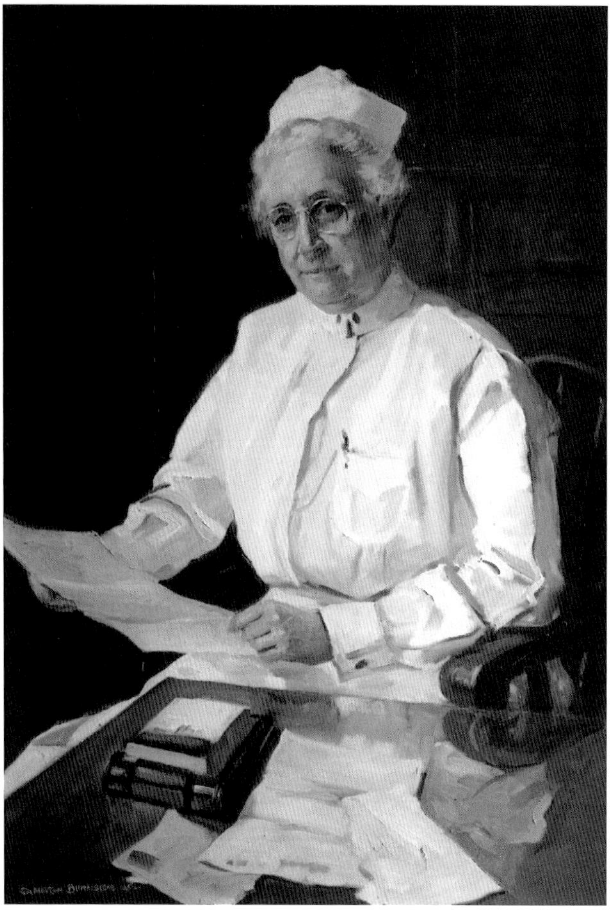

Left: A portrait of Helen G. McClelland, director of the Pennsylvania Hospital School of Nursing, 1933–56. *Courtesy of the Pennsylvania Hospital, Philadelphia, PAH Image Collection.*

Below: Nurses leaving Broad Street station, January 1942. *Courtesy of the Pennsylvania Hospital, Philadelphia, PAH School of Nursing Collection MG 3.13 ff5, Helen McClelland scrapbook.*

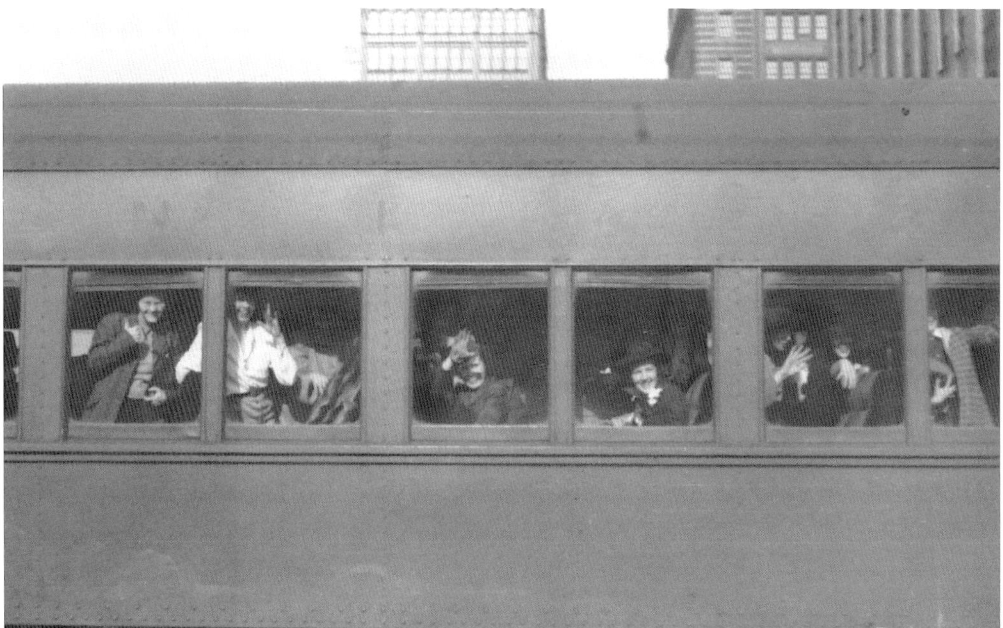

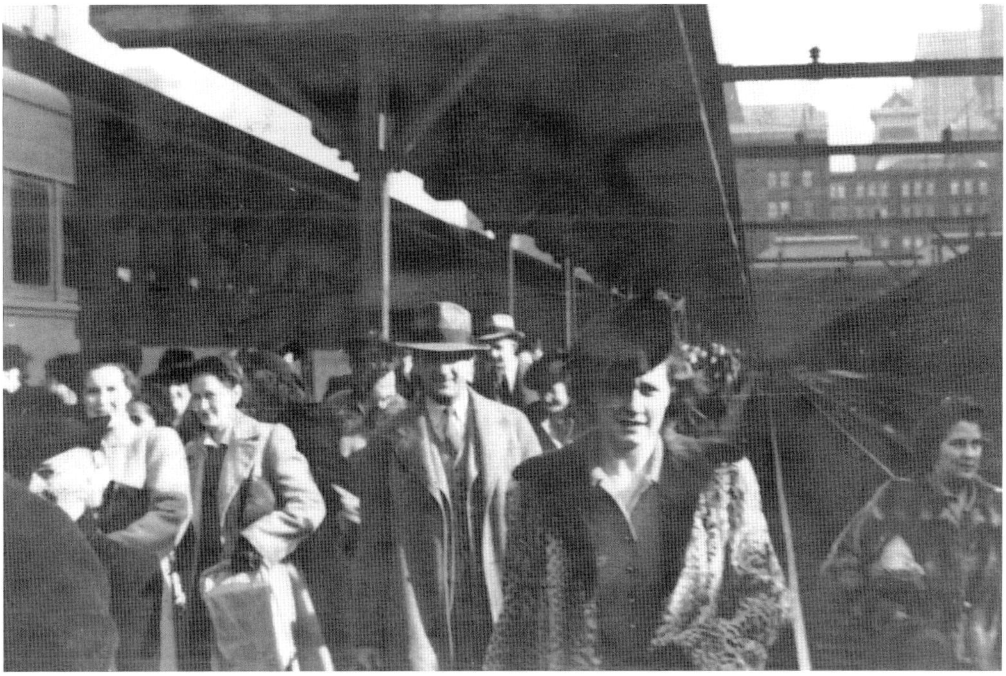

Nurses leaving Broad Street station, January 1942. *Courtesy of the Pennsylvania Hospital, Philadelphia, PAH School of Nursing Collection MG 3.13 ff5, Helen McClelland scrapbook.*

hospitals to prepare nurses. Federal money provided tuition, support for expansion and uniforms for nurses.

Ann Pekarik Stasheff came to Pennsylvania Hospital in 1945 as part of the program. She and her classmates wore hand-me-down nurses' uniforms as part of a war conservation effort, but their smart gray Cadet Corps uniforms were a point of pride, worn when they were outside of the hospital. Stasheff, who worked as a Pennsylvania Hospital operating room nurse for a few years after she graduated from the program, was proud to help the war effort. "So many of the staff had gone overseas, and there was rather a shortage in nursing," Stasheff remembers. "There were times that there would be only a graduate nurse on the floor, and so students were looking after an entire ward."

During the daytime, a head nurse was always present, but after 7:00 p.m., the students were largely responsible for the patients. Still, the quality of care remained high, Stasheff says. "As people came in, if they needed help, there was no question they got help. It didn't matter how much they could pay—a quarter, fifty cents."[104] Though the cadets and other volunteers served admirably, Hatfield said the hospital was glad to welcome back its returning doctors and nurses.[105]

THE BENJAMIN FRANKLIN CLINIC

In 1948, forty-four Pennsylvania Hospital physicians established the Benjamin Franklin Clinic, a new part of the hospital. The founders had all worked together in the Fifty-second Evacuation Unit during World War II, and during their time overseas they had come up with the plan for the clinic. It was a novel idea—focusing on preventive care and charging patients a flat fee for a complete diagnostic workup. The clinic took patients referred by their private physicians and represented a trend toward group practice. One of the founding physicians, Dr. Alexander Rush, a direct descendant of Dr. Benjamin Rush, would later become medical director of the clinic.

The clinic performed diagnostic and pre-placement tests, catering mostly to business and industrial firms and their executives. Patients paid one all-inclusive fee ($150 at the clinic's inception, with an average appointment stretching over four days or more), and for the doctors—all of whom were on the medical or surgical staff of the hospital—the clinic represented a chance to share costs and offer each other diagnostic and consultation services. Group practices were rare in that era, particularly in conservative Philadelphia; the famed Mayo Clinic was a Western phenomenon.[106]

The clinic often partnered with businesses, promising that the conservation of the health of executives was good for company balance sheets, and it gained attention for this focus on executives.[107] Some patients were so impressed by the clinic's services that they stayed on as permanent patients of the various doctors. As the cost of healthcare rose and companies became more aware that preventing health problems was cheaper than treating them, the clinic flourished. But by the 1970s, the clinic's business model had become outdated. "It was a fine innovation, and over time, because of costs rising, it became impractical. They did raise the fee, but it wasn't enough," said Dr. Robert Gill, a hospital physician for more than forty years who spent time working at the clinic early in his career.[108] The clinic existed in modified form—no more flat-fee services—until 2001, when it merged with the University of Pennsylvania Health System's Clinical Care Associates, a primary and specialty care network with various locations.

OBSTETRICS AND GYNECOLOGY

In the early twenty-first century, the obstetrics unit stands as one of Pennsylvania Hospital's busiest departments; the hospital is the most popular birthplace in Philadelphia, with nearly 5,000 babies born here a year. Between 1765 and 2007, more than 265,000 babies were born at the hospital. But the hospital's obstetrics unit might never have come into being if the founders had their say. The early managers never intended for babies to be born at Pennsylvania Hospital. Respectable women gave birth to their children at home, and, the managers reasoned, having a maternity ward would signal the board's tacit approval of immoral behavior. They were also against the idea of a foundling asylum, felt to be a necessary adjunct. Moreover, the medical profession did not yet recognize the need for separate maternity departments. Still, some maternity cases were accepted, and on July 17, 1765, one Martha Robinson, "a poor patient," delivered the first baby to be born at Pennsylvania Hospital.

It was not until a half century after the hospital's founding that a maternity department was established. In April 1793, the legislature set forth provisions for the establishment of a lying-in, or maternity, division at Pennsylvania Hospital. But another decade passed before these provisions were acted upon. The first child, a girl, was born at the Lying-in Department on April 27, 1803.

In 1803, obstetricians became the first specialists to be recognized at the hospital. In June 1810, at the managers' annual election of physicians and surgeons, separate lying-in doctors were elected. Thomas Chalkey James and John Moore were the first to hold the title. Dr. James, who is credited with the first successful induction of labor in 1810, was the first chairman of the department.[109] "Puerperal fever," also known as "childbed fever," or an infection of the genital tract shortly after birth, closed the Lying-in Department for the first time in late 1830. The department was reopened the next autumn after a thorough cleaning, but it closed again in 1854, following another puerperal fever attack that killed many patients in the department.[110]

Though the hospital itself no longer had a Lying-in Department, affiliations with other lying-in facilities continued. One such facility was the Philadelphia Lying-in Charity for Attending Indigent Women in their own Home, which was founded in 1828. It allied itself with the Philadelphia Nurse Society, which, in part, trained obstetric nurses, and in 1863 it became known as the Philadelphia Lying-in Charity and Nurse Society. In 1923, the organization joined forces with Pennsylvania Hospital, a natural move since many of the managers of the hospital were also managers of the Lying-in Charity. The State Hospital for Women and Infants, chartered in 1872 and later known simply as the Maternity Hospital, also associated with Pennsylvania Hospital in 1930. A main purpose of this organization was to offer "unfortunate" women privacy and a chance for social readjustment; it was also a training site for many nurses.

In 1960, a final maternity affiliation was made, this time with the Preston Retreat, so named for Dr. Jonas Preston, Philadelphia philanthropist, whose will endowed a fund to aid "indigent married women of good character." Dr. Preston was born in 1764 in Chester, Pennsylvania, and graduated from the University of Pennsylvania's School of Medicine. He served as a member of the Pennsylvania legislature, where he authored the law that granted all children free public education. He also served on city council, where he helped promote the construction of a waterworks for the city. Dr. Preston died in 1836 and willed $250,000 for the Preston Retreat. In 1837, the cornerstone was laid in a section of the city between Second and Third Streets and Hamilton and Schuylkill Streets. The retreat opened in 1866—the managers opted to not open until they lightened their debt load—and on February 6, 1866, Jane Preston Hynes, named for the founder, was born. Mortality rates were low, and the average patient stayed at the retreat for thirty days. A school of midwifery and practical nursing was opened at the retreat in 1916.[111]

The Preston Retreat had shared services with Pennsylvania Hospital prior to their formal affiliation, and so the partnership seemed a natural one, although Preston

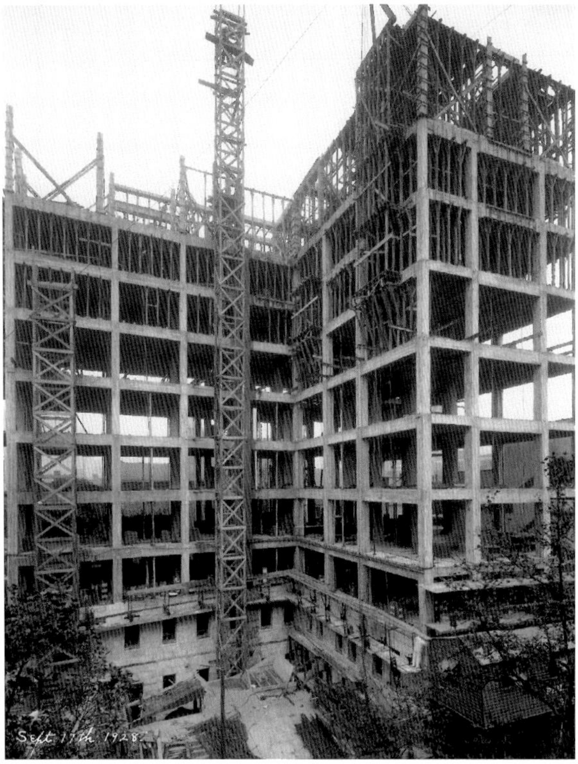

The Spruce Building, at Eighth and Spruce Streets, under construction. *Courtesy of the Pennsylvania Hospital, Philadelphia, PAH Image Collection 223.*

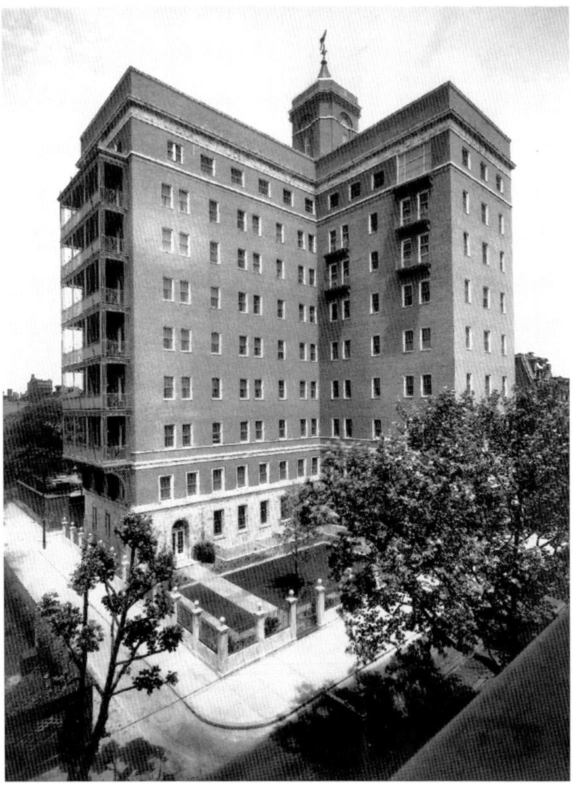

The completed Spruce Building, 1929. *Courtesy of the Pennsylvania Hospital, Philadelphia, PAH Image Collection 200a.*

did consider joining with other area hospitals.[112] Another obstetrical milestone was achieved in 1964, when staff physician Edward H. Bishop published the first scientific criteria for elective induction of labor. Obstetricians everywhere are now familiar with the "Bishop score."[113]

In 1971, the Preston Building opened at Pennsylvania Hospital through another bequest of Dr. Preston. Previously, the lying-in facilities were housed in the Spruce Building. Since the opening of the Preston Building, the hospital has become known for its cutting-edge innovations and top-notch obstetrical care. In 1978, the region's first antenatal testing unit, or ATU, was founded to diagnose and evaluate the fetus.

In 1985, the first GIFT, or gamete intrafallopian transfer, pregnancy was achieved in the city. Pennsylvania Hospital's GIFT program was one of the first of its kind in the United States. A decade later, Pennsylvania Hospital had seen one thousand live births from GIFT and other reproductive technologies. The first laparoscopic-assisted vaginal hysterectomy in the city was performed at the hospital in 1985. And in 1996, the hospital opened the region's first perinatal evaluation and treatment unit, or PETU, to assist

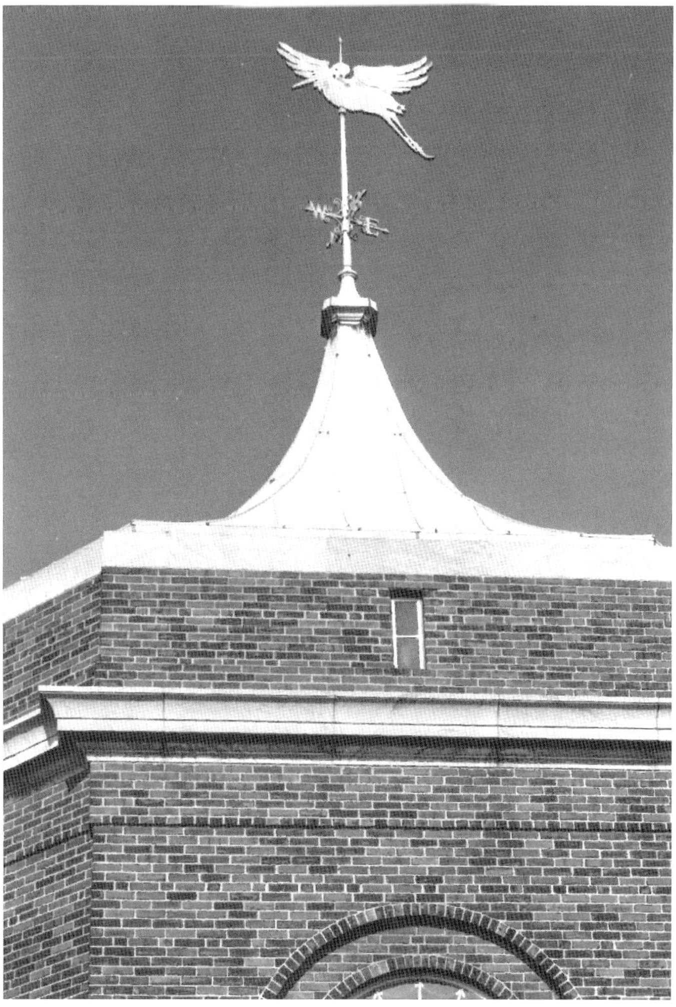

The cupola of the Women's Building (now Spruce Building) with its stork weathervane. The Birthing Suite, located in the Spruce Building, is available to women experiencing low-risk pregnancies who opt for low- or no-intervention labor with the assistance of a certified nurse-midwife. *Courtesy of the Pennsylvania Hospital, Philadelphia, PAH Image Collection 408.*

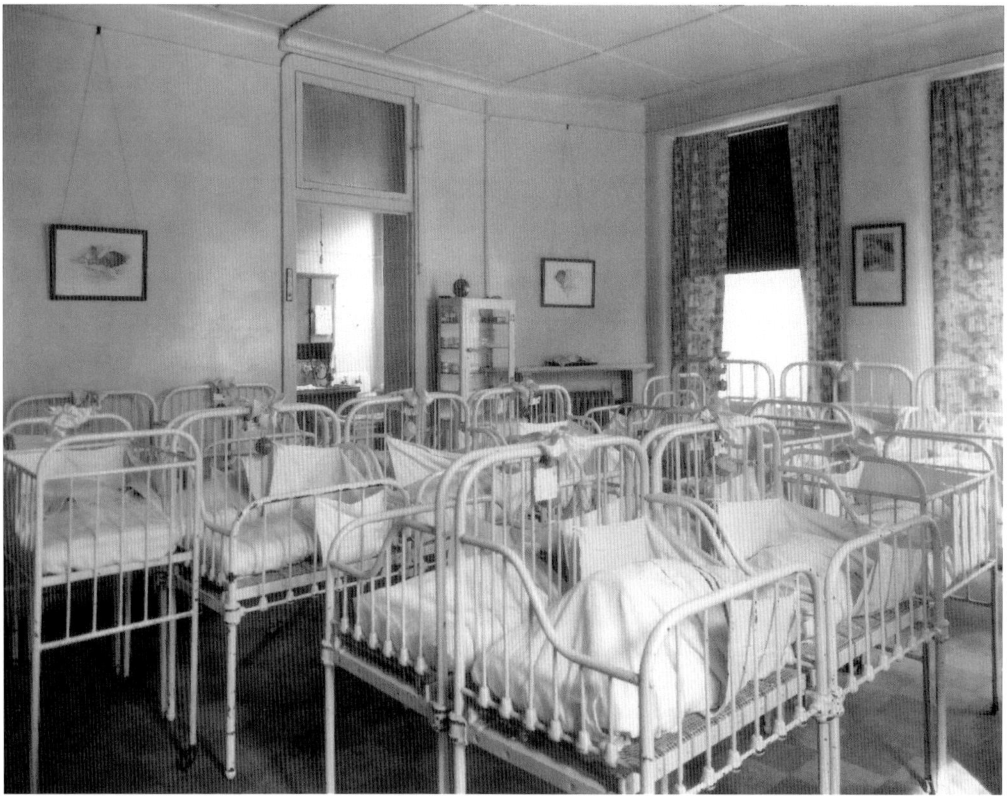

A 1929 image of a ward nursery in the Women's Building (currently the Spruce Building). *Courtesy of the Pennsylvania Hospital, Philadelphia, PAH Image Collection 773.*

in the evaluation of high-risk situations that develop during labor. Procedures such as amniocentesis and fetal surgery are also performed in the PETU.

A large percentage of the infants born at Pennsylvania Hospital come from high-risk pregnancies, and the hospital's neonatology department remains, as it has been since the 1950s, at the forefront of patient care. The neonatal team is known for its successful care of extremely small infants, some weighing less than five hundred grams, or one pound. According to data from an international comparative database, Pennsylvania Hospital consistently ranks among the best centers in the country for preterm infants. The hospital offers a full range of "alternative birthing" options as well, including the Birthing Suite at Pennsylvania Hospital, which allows expectant mothers to choose low- or no-intervention births minutes away from state-of-the-art obstetrical care. Mothers can also choose to be treated by a certified nurse-midwife—an experienced registered nurse educated and certified in midwifery. These professions provide prenatal care, deliver babies and offer regular gynecologic care for healthy women with uncomplicated pregnancies. Nurse-midwives focus on education and personal attention.[114]

WOMEN IN MEDICINE AT PENNSYLVANIA HOSPITAL

In 1869, the board of managers granted permission for students from the Women's Medical College of Philadelphia to join with male students at the hospital. The school, first known as "Female Medical College of Pennsylvania," was incorporated in 1850. It was the first of several institutions in the country devoted solely to the medical education of women. On November 6, about thirty women entered Pennsylvania Hospital's amphitheatre to hisses and catcalls from the male students. Soon after, the board of managers passed a resolution censuring the behavior of the male students, a move that gained attention in the local newspapers.

Public sentiment was stirred, with medical professionals generally opposed to the managers' action. At a meeting on November 16, 1869, the faculties of both the University of Pennsylvania and the Jefferson Medical College, and members of a number of hospital staffs, signed a petition to keep women out of the clinics. The fervor continued until 1871, when the contributors to Pennsylvania Hospital passed a resolution requiring the members of the staff to teach women. Some members of the staff decided to give one lecture a week to women in addition to their regular semiweekly lectures to men. Dr. D. Hayes Agnew was so strongly opposed to teaching women that he declined to be named surgeon at the hospital. But eventually he changed his mind and even lectured to mixed classes.

NURSING AT PENNSYLVANIA HOSPITAL

The history of nursing at Pennsylvania Hospital effectively began in 1752, when it was announced that the hospital would accept patients and that "a suitable matron to take care of the house and of the Sick" had been hired. Elizabeth Gardner, a Quaker widow, served from November 6, 1751, to May 14, 1760. Gardner's work was esteemed by the hospital, as evident in this note from Benjamin Franklin: "Sister Elizabeth, Please to receive the Bearer into the Hospital, & entertain him there till the Physicians have considered his Case. Your Friend & Serv, B. Franklin."[115] In the early records of the manager's minutes, it is noted that Alice Courtnet joined the staff as maid and nurse.[116]

There was not yet formal training for nurses in those days—a woman or man who bore the title of nurse was simply one who was willing to care for the ill and infirm.[117] Nurses were often plucked from the ranks of the former patients, those who had shown interest and aptitude for the job and were generally trustworthy. Some were taken from other jobs and put into nursing ranks. In 1796, Elizabeth Truby was hired as housemaid; she spent a year as a nurse, and then, in 1799, she again became a nurse. Elizabeth Brown,

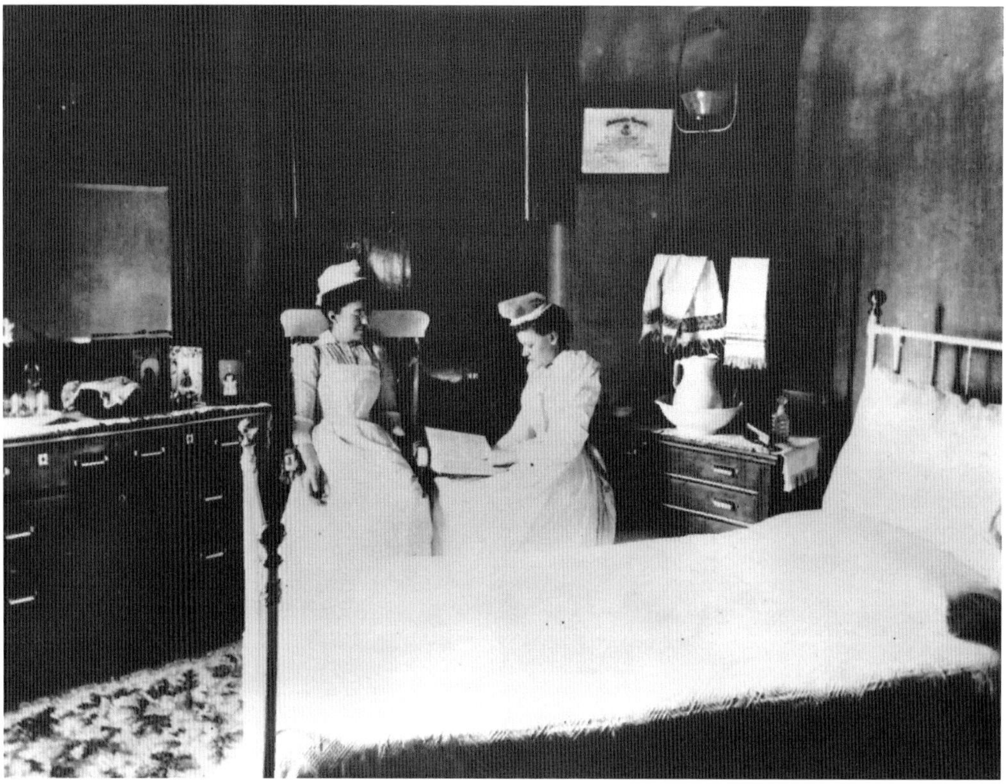

An 1887 image of a nurses bedroom with two nurses seated. *Courtesy of the Pennsylvania Hospital, Philadelphia, PAH Image Collection 619b.*

Pennsylvania Hospital cowherd, became assistant nurse in 1788. Catherine Burns and Ruth Carrigan, who were hospital cooks, also became nurses.[118] These nurses were often members of the working poor, with little education. There is scant mention of early nursing arrangements among the hospital's archives, but one allusion to "experienced and trustworthy persons" was made. Responsibilities were not spelled out in records, but likely included carrying food, tending fires, bathing patients, emptying vessels, handling dressings, quieting disturbances and even burying the dead. For this work, they were paid between eight and twenty pounds a year in the hospital's earliest days.[119]

By 1800, the hospital employed a nurse for each of the two sick wards—men's and women's—a nurse for venereal patients housed in the former apothecary building and a "nurse of the cells." At least two assistant nurses were also employed. Nursing turnover, which was high in the colonial era, lessened, and some nurses became known for their skill. One, nurse Kitty Burns, became particularly expert in laying out the dead, a task that paid extra.[120] Later in the nineteenth century, around 1864, women visitors were permitted into the male wards, but they were only allowed in to perform such "harmless" duties as reading aloud religious material.[121]

In 1875, the managers considered a plan to establish a training school for nurses. A program was developed, including medical and surgical components. Applicants

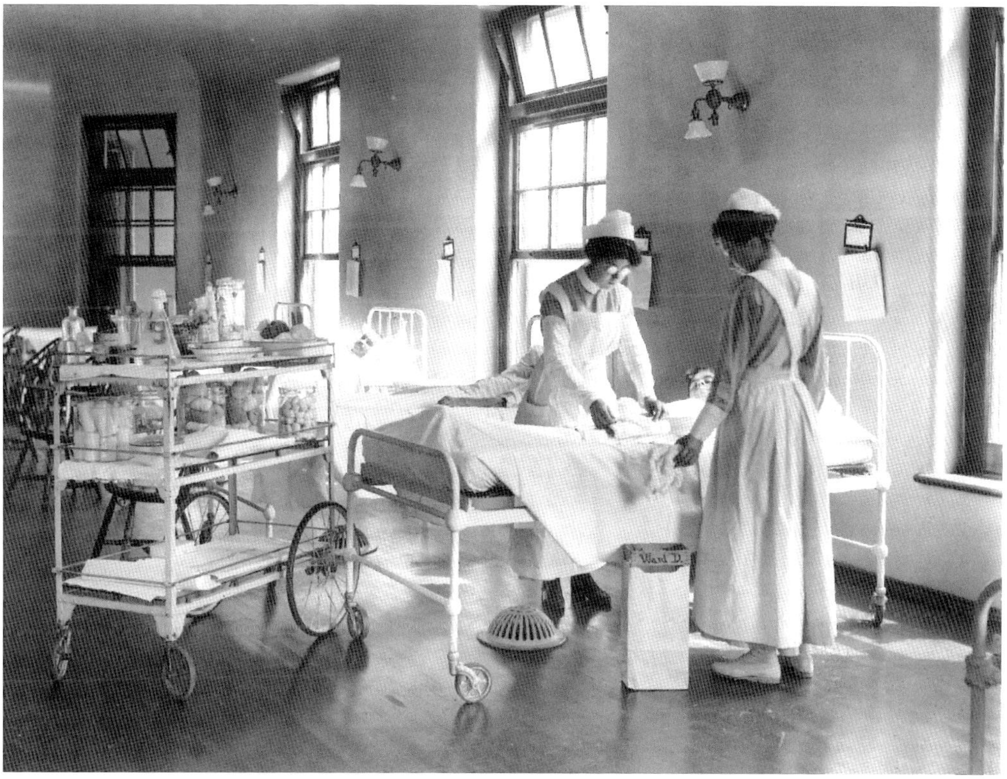

Nurses collecting soiled bandages from a patient, circa 1900. *Courtesy of the Pennsylvania Hospital, Philadelphia, PAH Image Collection.*

had to be twenty-one, and once a candidate finished the coursework, she received a certificate if she "fulfilled all the requirements of the course and showed good conduct and competency in nursing." Four years later, the hospital made an agreement with the Women's Hospital of Philadelphia to co-train their student nurses. It was a partnership that lasted until 1882. An independent nurses' school was reestablished in 1883, with four nurses graduated that first year. Temporary quarters were built for the nursing students in the Picture House—the structure built in 1818 to house the Benjamin West painting *Christ Healing the Sick in the Temple*—which was outfitted for the nurses for about $4,500.

Members of the medical, surgical and outpatient staffs delivered lectures to the student nurses, supplementing instruction by the school's superintendent. The high quality of education in the school led to a new way of staffing the hospital. In 1885, three female nurses were permitted to work on the men's medical wards. Previously, only men could work on these wards. The nursing course was extended to two years, and in 1897, to three. The first public commencement of nurses occurred in 1893, when students received pins that bore the seal of the Good Samaritan on the design. It was also that year that a new "Nurses' Home" was completed on the hospital's grounds. The three-story building cost $50,000 to construct.[122]

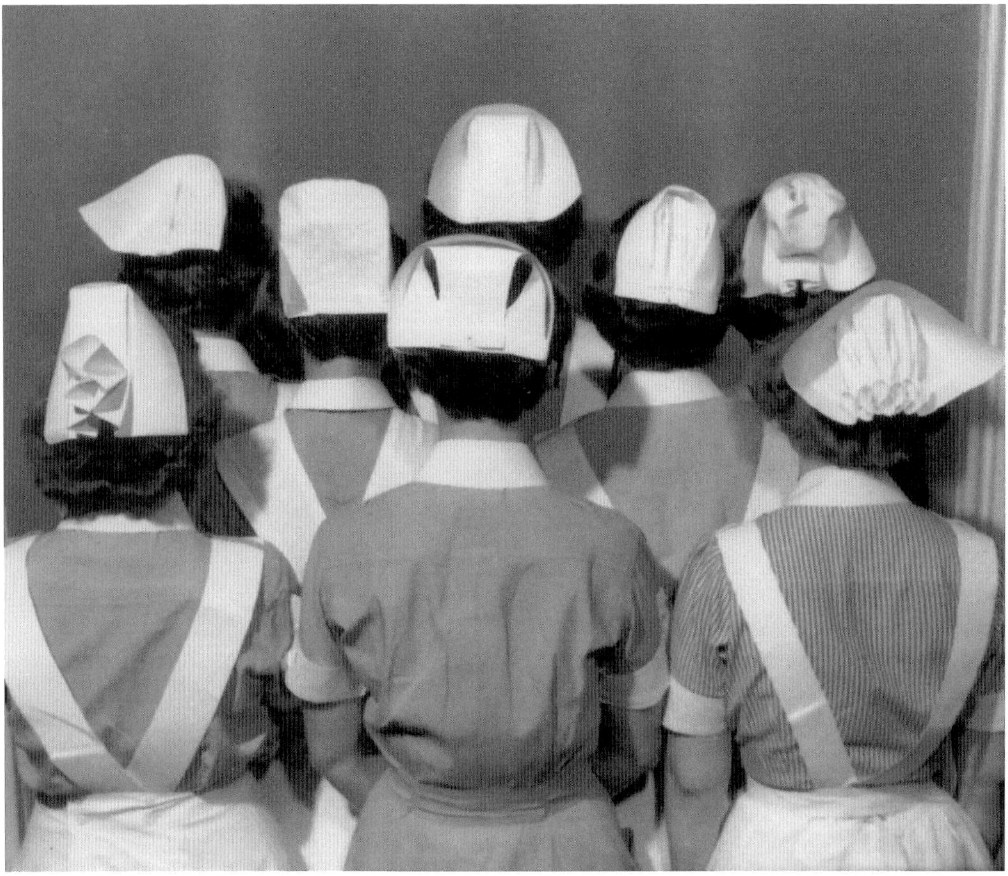

Many early caps were made of muslin or organdy; some had elaborate frills. By 1910, simpler caps came into use. At Pennsylvania Hospital, a stiff-brimmed, highly starched rear ruffle remained in use. *Courtesy of the Pennsylvania Hospital, Philadelphia, PAH Image Collection.*

One of the most distinguished members of the nursing training school was Miss Lucy Walker, an English nurse who became superintendent in 1895. Walker is considered one of the early leaders in the development of professional nursing in America. She reorganized the training school, started the Nurses Alumnae Association and was a founder of the Philadelphia County Nurses Association, the American Journal of Nursing Company, and the Associated Alumnae of the United States, a forerunner to the American Nurses Association. She was one of the first teachers in the nursing course started at the Teacher's College at Columbia University in 1900,[123] and she also helped establish the American Society of Superintendents of Training Schools for Nurses, a forerunner to the National League for Nursing.[124] Her guidance led the school to become recognized as one of the best in the United States. Miss Margaret A. Dunlop, who took over the school in 1909, helped organize the American Ambulance Service and Base Hospital No. 10 during World War I. An assistant, Miss Helen G. McClelland, received the American Distinguished Service Cross for her valorous service during World War I, and she succeeded Dunlop.

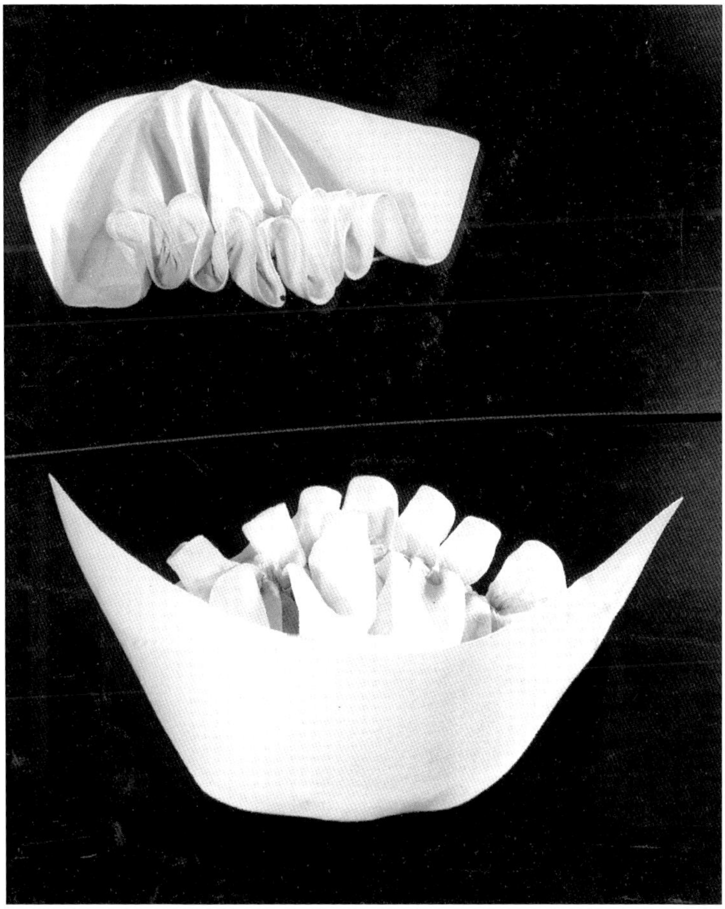

A close-up view of a Pennsylvania Hospital nurses cap. *Courtesy of the Pennsylvania Hospital, Philadelphia, PAH Image Collection 1657b.*

McClelland oversaw the school for twenty-three years, during which time the dynamics of the nursing profession changed tremendously. She brought a shorter work day for nurses, encouraged continuing education, designed nursing education programs and encouraged friends of the hospital to endow scholarships. McClelland also organized the nursing end of the Fifty-second Evacuation Hospital during World War II.[125] Ann Pekarik Stasheff was a student in the nursing program during World War II, and she remembers McClelland fondly. "She could be stern, but as a person she was warm and caring," Stasheff says. "She was the ideal nursing director— she helped the hospital move ahead and worked extremely well with the administration. They did a great deal in promoting the hospital to where it is now from where it had been." Even in her retirement, McClelland still connected with her former students and nurses. She retired to Pennsylvania Dutch country and invited her nurses to visit her. Stasheff did so and remembers a quilt that McClelland displayed proudly, a creation of old nurses' uniforms stitched together.[126]

In 1914, Dr. Owen Copp established the School of Nursing for Men at Pennsylvania Hospital. (It was the first nursing school for males in the country that was led by a man, Leroy N. Craig.) The school provided generalized training, combined with specialization in psychiatric and urological nursing. An Affiliate Program in Psychiatric Nursing was established in 1932, and the School of Nursing for Men was one of just nine hospital-based nursing schools to participate in this cooperative program. During the 1950s, Craig and Congresswoman Frances Payne Bolton ensured that male nurses were granted commissions in the armed forces, and several graduates of Pennsylvania Hospital's school were among the first to enter.

The School of Nursing for Men operated until 1965, when changes in accreditation and administration made it more practical to merge the School of Nursing for Men at Forty-ninth Street with the School of Nursing for Women at Eighth Street. Nursing education was changing—while the hospital's programs had been based on the "diploma school" format, with clinical experience and classroom instruction playing roles, there was now more pressure to create a more academic school. The faculty of the new, merged program updated their curriculum based on the new trends in nursing education. However, in 1974, economic pressures and those new trends in preparing nurses forced the closure of both the School of Nursing and the Affiliate Program in Psychiatric Nursing at the Institute.

"It was a most difficult decision," H. Robert Cathcart, president of the hospital, said at the time. "We agonized over it for months. After all, this school has a distinguished and illustrious history, and you just can't close its doors without some intense soul-searching. But the hard facts of a budget that will not stretch any further, plus the very serious questions of the future of hospital programs, finally made the decision for us." In all, Pennsylvania Hospital trained nearly three thousand nurses.[127]

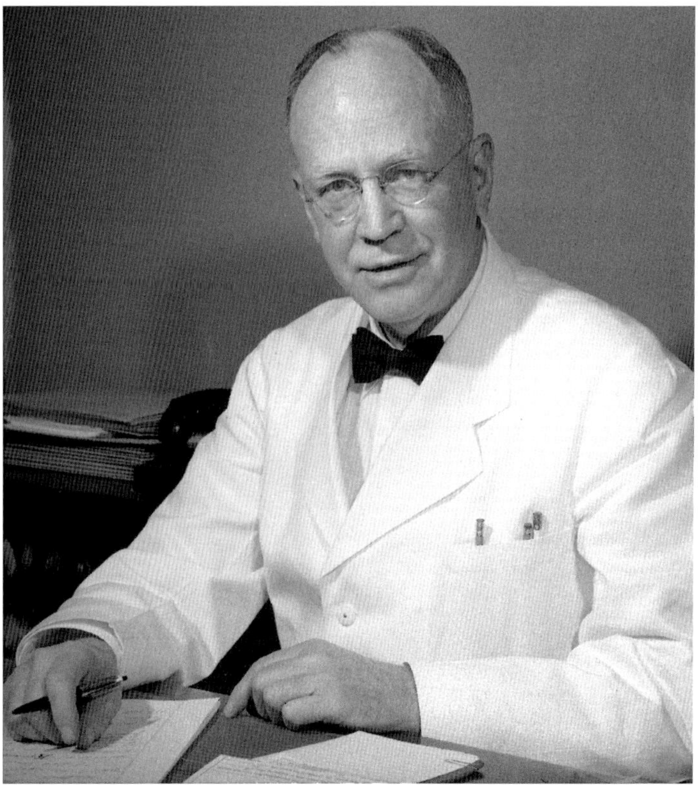

A portrait of LeRoy Craig, director of the Pennsylvania Hospital School of Nursing for Men, from 1914 through 1956. *Courtesy of the Pennsylvania Hospital, Philadelphia; PAH School of Nursing Collection, MG 3.14 ff1.*

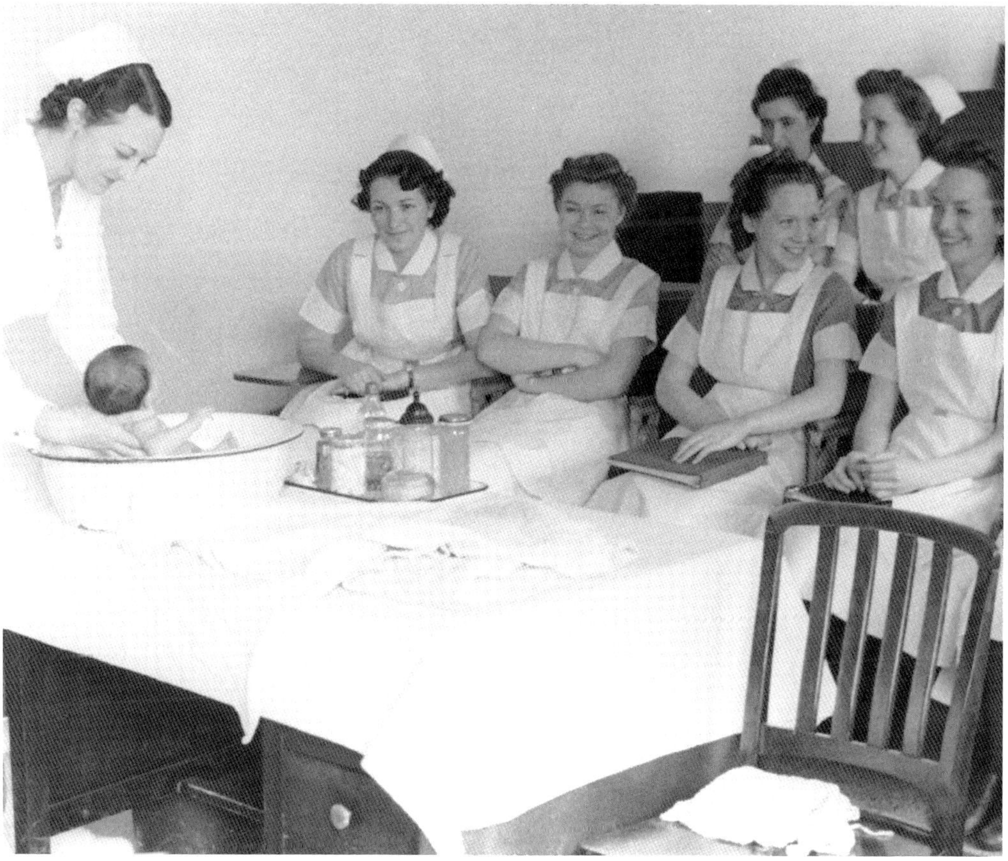

A 1930s maternity nursing class. *Courtesy of the Pennsylvania Hospital, Philadelphia, PAH Image Collection.*

In 1979, the book *Nurse* by Peggy Anderson made a splash in the publishing world. It was based on the story of a head nurse at Pennsylvania Hospital, and it spent weeks atop the *New York Times* bestseller list. Anderson had spent months researching the lives of nurses and ended up centering on a nurse she called Mary Benjamin. The book, which was made into a television show, received critical acclaim. Anderson said that she wrote the book because she felt that the nurse's was "a story that had never been told. Virtually all popular versions of the world of medicine have starred doctors." She painted nurses as playing a crucial role in the hospital and in patient care, and said that setting the book at Pennsylvania Hospital was ideal because the hospital was "a place where nurses are encouraged to explore their full range as professionals, and where nurses are supported."[128]

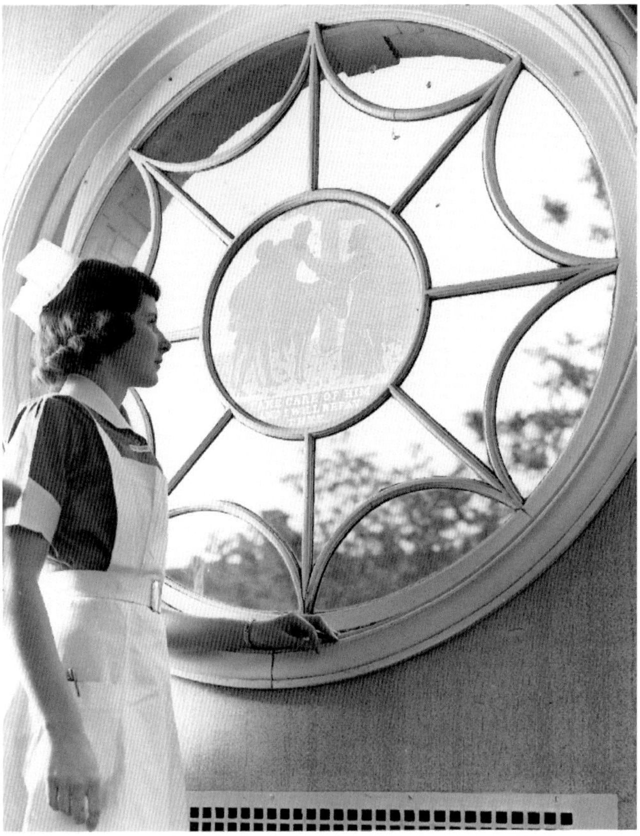

Left: A 1954 image of a nurse looking out a window with the Good Samaritan Seal etched in the center glass. *Courtesy of the Pennsylvania Hospital, Philadelphia, PAH Image Collection 1618.*

Below: A 1942 capping ceremony. Nurse Helen McClelland pins caps on recent graduate nurses. *Courtesy of the Pennsylvania Hospital, Philadelphia, PAH Image Collection 1281.*

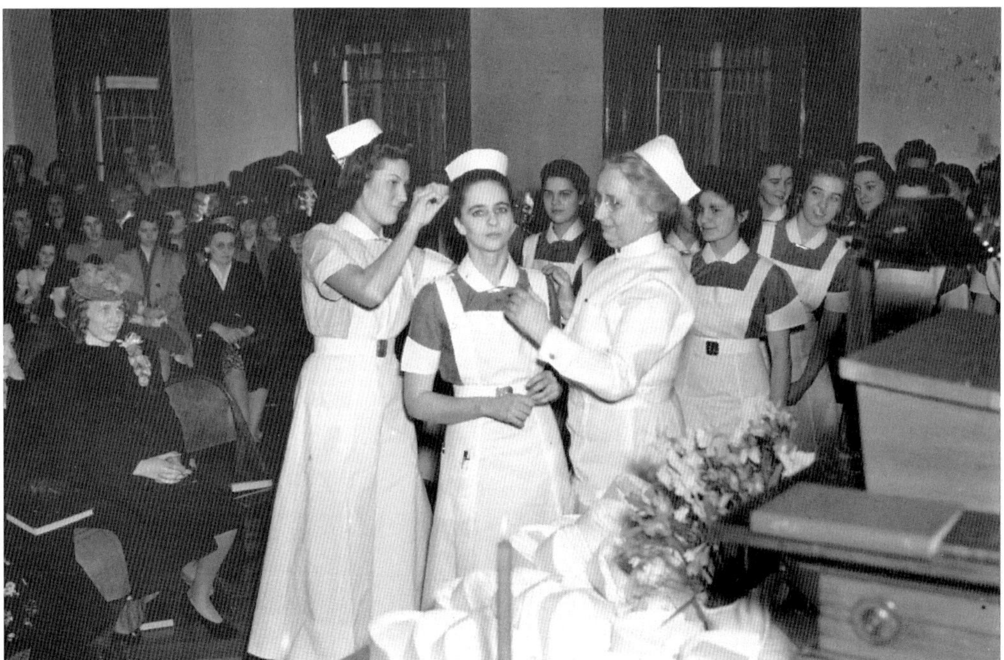

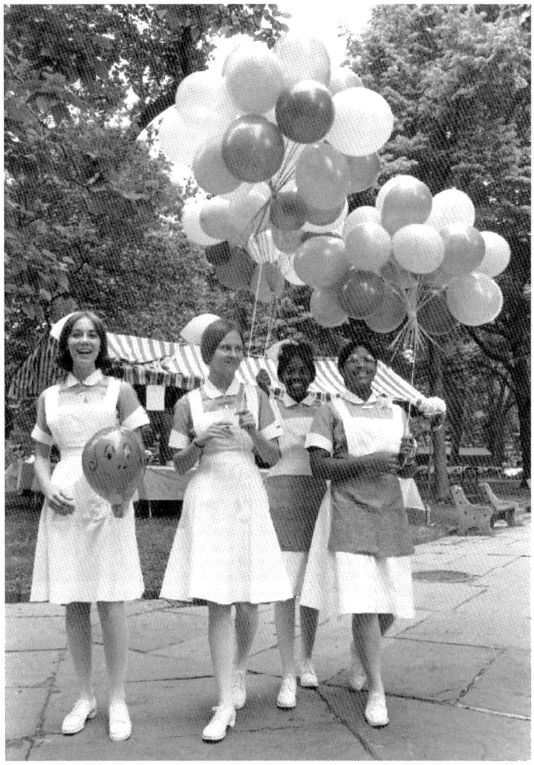

Right: A 1970 Pennsylvania Hospital Day celebration. *Courtesy of the Pennsylvania Hospital, Philadelphia, PAH Image Collection.*

Below: Nurse Ann Louise Devenney at the nurse's station. *Courtesy of the Pennsylvania Hospital, Philadelphia, PAH Image Collection.*

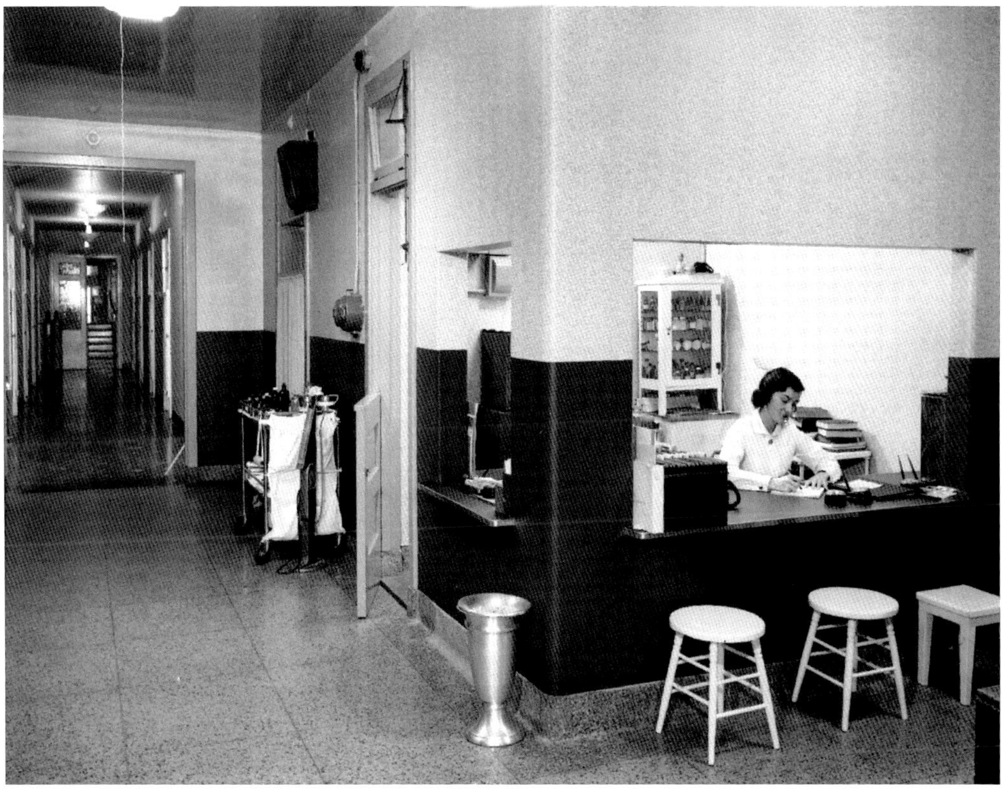

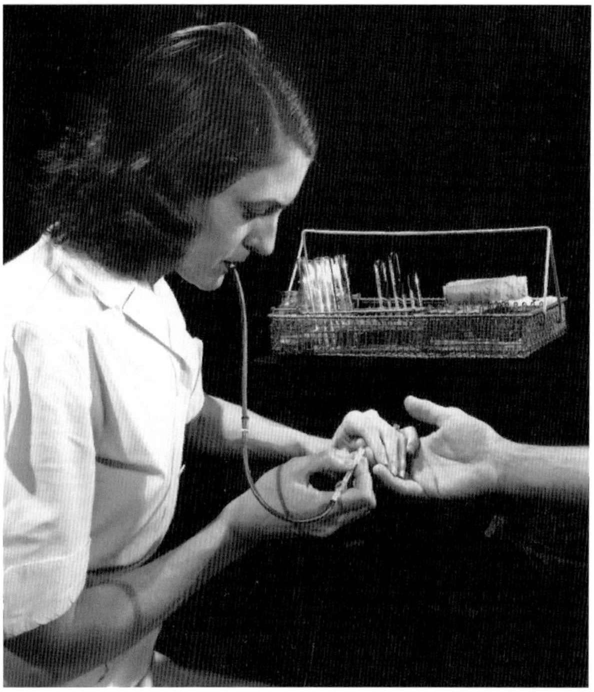

Left: A nurse drawing blood (1950s). *Courtesy of the Pennsylvania Hospital, Philadelphia, PAH Image Collection.*

Below: A nurse with glass vials (1950s). *Courtesy of the Pennsylvania Hospital, Philadelphia, PAH Image Collection.*

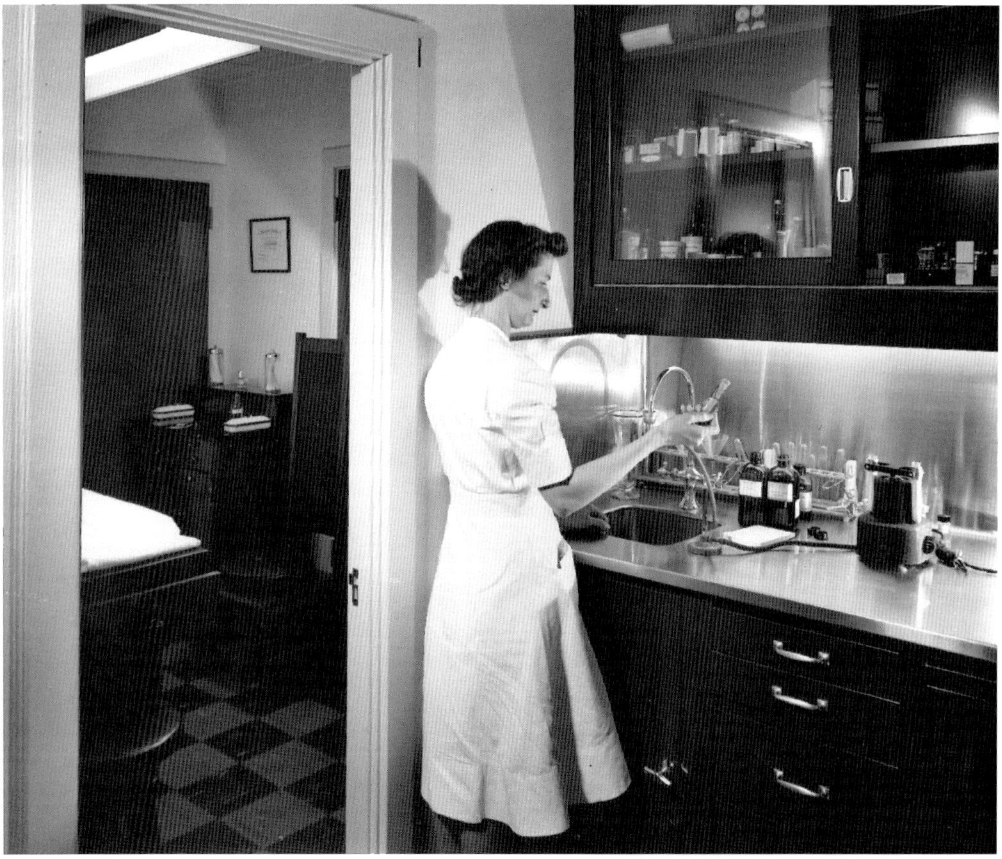

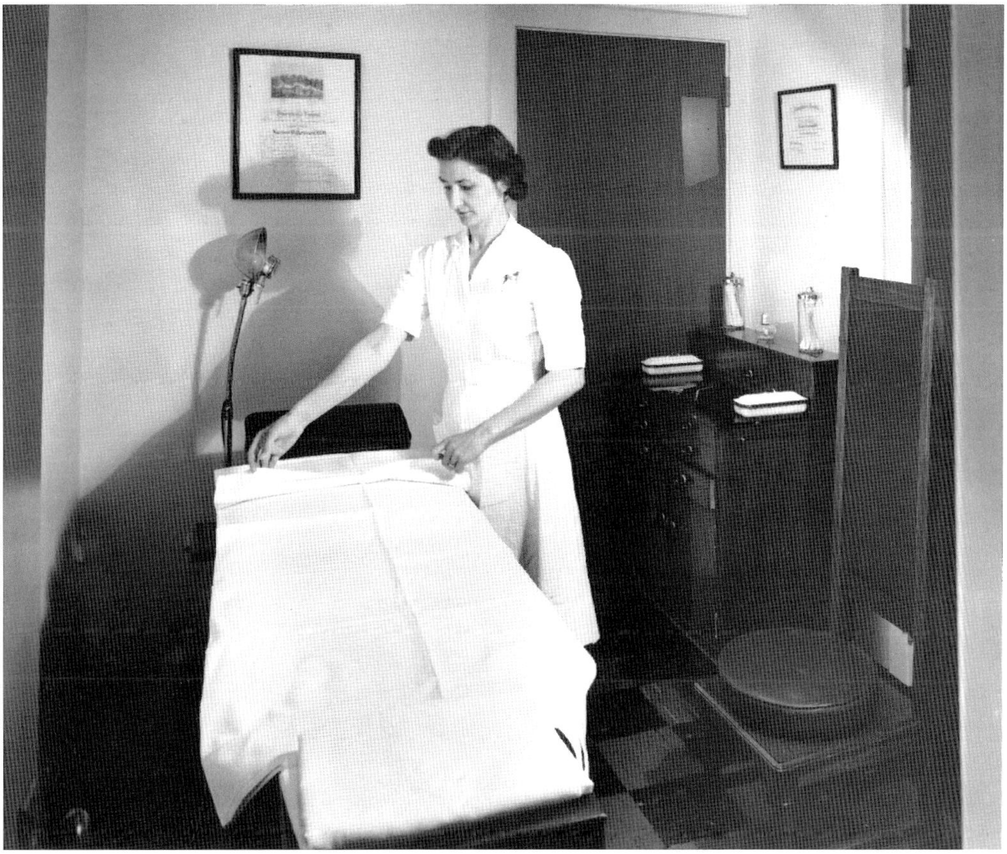

A nurse repairing an exam room (1950s). *Courtesy of the Pennsylvania Hospital, Philadelphia, PAH Image Collection.*

BUILDINGS, ARTWORK AND GROUNDS

The contemporary hospital is a Center City campus made up of several buildings and bounded by Seventh and Ninth Streets and Pine and Locust Streets. The original hospital structure, the Pine Building, a Federal-style brick and stone structure, is still a thriving part of the campus today, housing mainly administrative offices and the medical library. In large part, the Pine Building exterior looks as it did in 1804, when its center section was finished. Its imposing Great Court, with Portuguese tile floor, and other rooms occupy the center section's floor. The wood-paneled Historic Library and the surgical amphitheatre are located on the second and third floors. About six thousand visitors a year walk through the Pine Building.

The hospital's signature piece of art is the Benjamin West painting *Christ Healing the Sick in the Temple*. West, who was born in Delaware County in 1792, was once historical painter to King George III. In 1800, the managers wrote to him inquiring whether he would consider painting a picture to donate to the hospital. West said he would, suggesting as the topic Christ healing the sick in the temple. The managers agreed, and

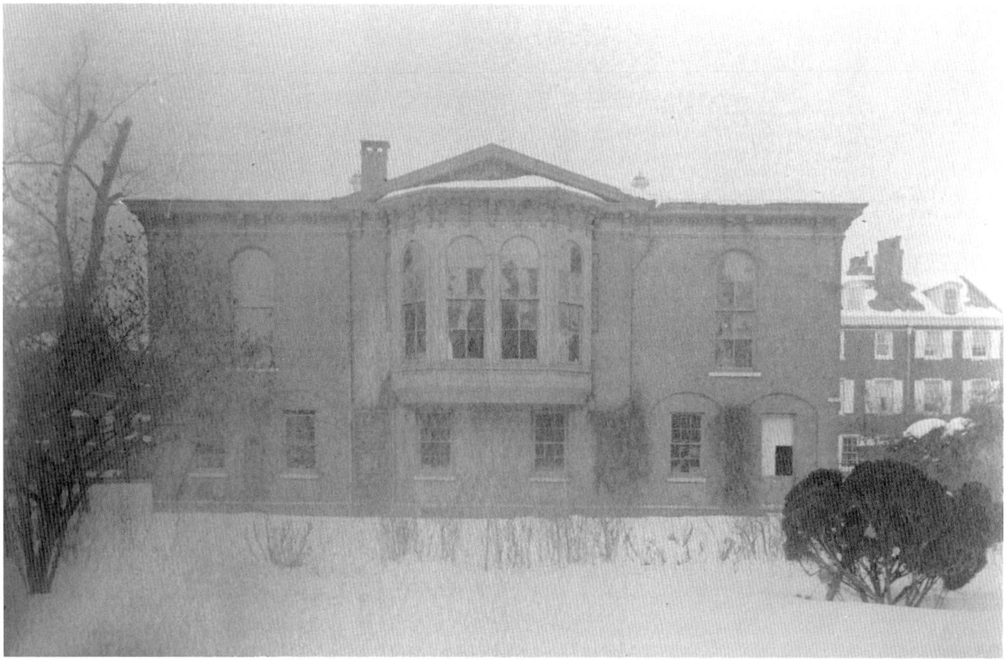

The Picture House (circa 1890s), originally built to house Benjamin West's painting of *Christ Healing the Sick in the Temple*. Later it was used as the nurses' residence. *Courtesy of the Pennsylvania Hospital, Philadelphia, PAH Image Collection 194.*

after several delays, West wrote, saying, "I have finished the picture of Our Saviour receiving the Lame and the Blind in the Temple to heal them, with that success, to render it in the judgment of our lovers of the arts as holding the first rank in my production of the pencil." He went on to explain that he had been pressured into selling it to officers of the British Institution for the proposed National Gallery for the sum of £3,000. He would paint a replica for the hospital, he promised, better than the first. He even added a "demoniac with his attendant relations," a nod to Pennsylvania Hospital's treatment of the mentally ill.

In 1817, it was finally finished, a gift to the hospital in memory of West's wife, Elizabeth, also a Philadelphia native. The managers decided that instead of hanging the work in their boardroom, as originally planned, they would erect a small building to house it. Beginning in 1818, after the work finally arrived in Philadelphia, the "Picture House" was home to West's work. The hospital charged admission for viewing the painting and gave all who visited a written description of *Christ Healing the Sick*. In all, about $15,000 was raised in the first year of exhibition—thirty thousand visitors came to see West's work. The painting was loaned to the Pennsylvania Academy of the Fine Arts several times, and for a time it was housed in the Institute before returning to the Eighth Street campus in 1884, when it was hung in the clinical amphitheatre. Since then, it has hung in the main part of the Pine Building, where visitors may still observe it today.[129]

In addition to West's work, the hospital has a rich collection of paintings and other objects. A Thomas Eakins portrait of Pennsylvania Hospital physician Dr. Jacob

DaCosta, a staff physician for many years, is a highlight. There are two original works by the renowned artist Thomas Sully—one is a portrait of Samuel Coates, an early member of the board of managers, and one is a portrait of Dr. Benjamin Rush. Sully donated the former as his gift to the hospital, and the second was purchased after a number of Dr. Rush's students asked that money from the Medical Fund be used for such a purpose following Dr. Rush's death.[130] There are also portraits of Jacob Ehrenzeller, the first medical apprentice in the country, and of Dr. Phillip Syng Physick, the father of American surgery.

Also on display at the hospital is an antique fire engine, purchased by the managers in 1803. It is believed to be the work of Philadelphia engine maker Philip Mason. It was bought so employees could pump their own water in case of fire, and the board was so enamored of the fire engine that they ordered it tested before each managers' meeting.[131] A large astronomical, musical clock made by David Rittenhouse (an astronomer, mathematician, surveyor, first Pennsylvania state treasurer and first director of the U.S. Mint) in about 1780 still sits in the Pine Building. The clock, which is said to have originally cost the astonishing sum of more than $1,000, was loaned to the hospital in 1819 by Sarah Zane and bequeathed to the hospital after her death in 1870.[132] The

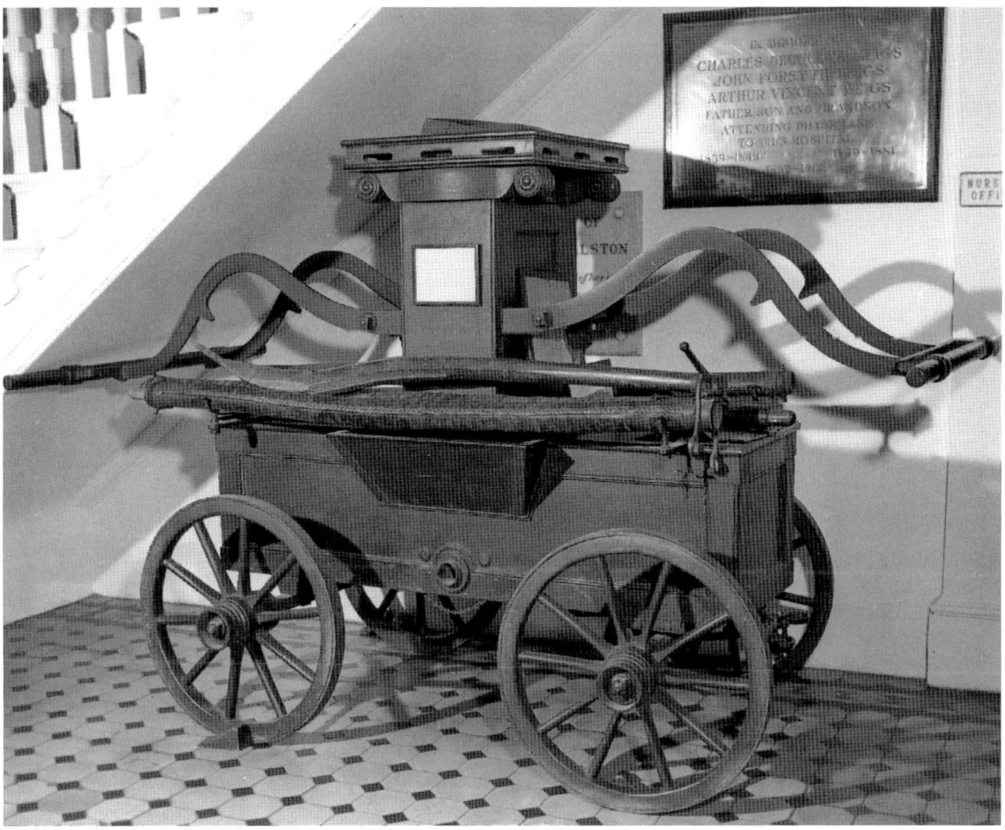

The fire engine purchased by the board of managers in 1803 to prevent fires from escalating and destroying the hospital. The fire engine is currently on view in the Great Court of the Pine Building. *Courtesy of the Pennsylvania Hospital, Philadelphia, PAH Image Collection 1656.*

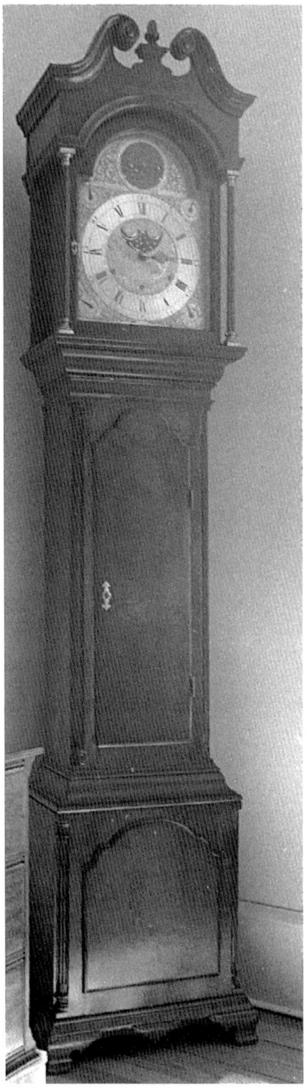

An image of the David Rittenhouse clock. The clock is currently on view in the Pine Building. *Courtesy of the Pennsylvania Hospital, Philadelphia, PAH Image Collection 1607.2.*

clock is considered by some to be one of the finest timepieces ever constructed, and after meetings of the board of managers, the gentlemen would retire to the clock. During one restoration of the timepiece, a bottle of Madeira was found in the bottom—it seems the men stored their post-meeting refreshments there. The Rittenhouse clock broke sometime in the 1960s, but in 1975, a six-year-long restoration was completed.[133]

Other historic objects owned by the hospital include a silver wine cooler that Chief Justice John Marshall presented to Dr. Phillip Syng Physick in 1831 after a successful operation, and a large, cast-lead statue of William Penn, which came to the hospital in 1804, having been purchased in a London junk shop by John Penn, William Penn's grandson. An old legend says that once a year, as the clock strikes midnight to usher in the New Year, William Penn descends from his perch to take a walk around the hospital grounds.[134]

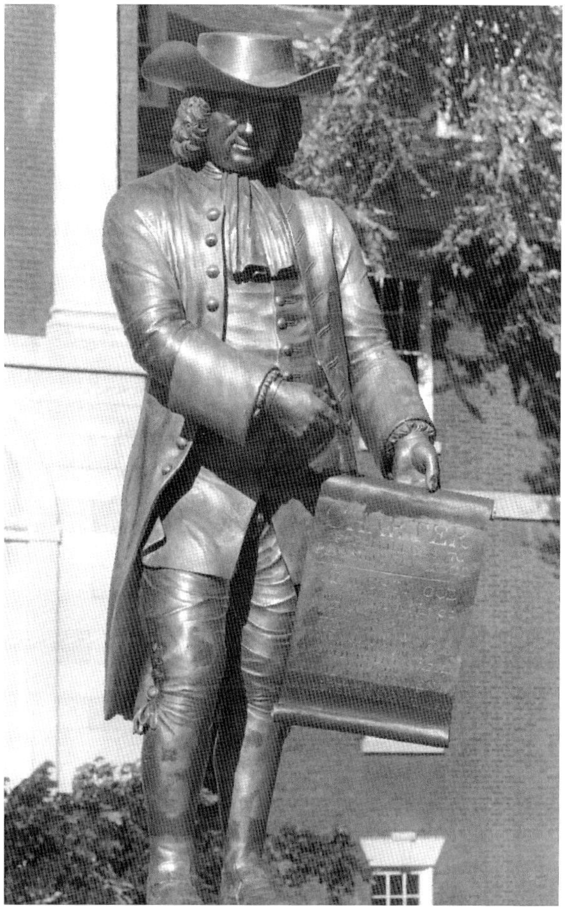

Right: The statue of William Penn after its restoration (1982). This statue has graced the front of the Pine Building since it was donated by John Penn in 1804. *Courtesy of the Pennsylvania Hospital, Philadelphia, PAH Image Collection.*

Below: A 1976 image of Physic Garden designer Martha Garra (left), with volunteers Cecily Clark (far right) and Sallie Harvey tending to trillium. Trillium was used in the eighteenth century to reduce fever. *Courtesy of the Pennsylvania Hospital, Philadelphia, PAH Image Collection.*

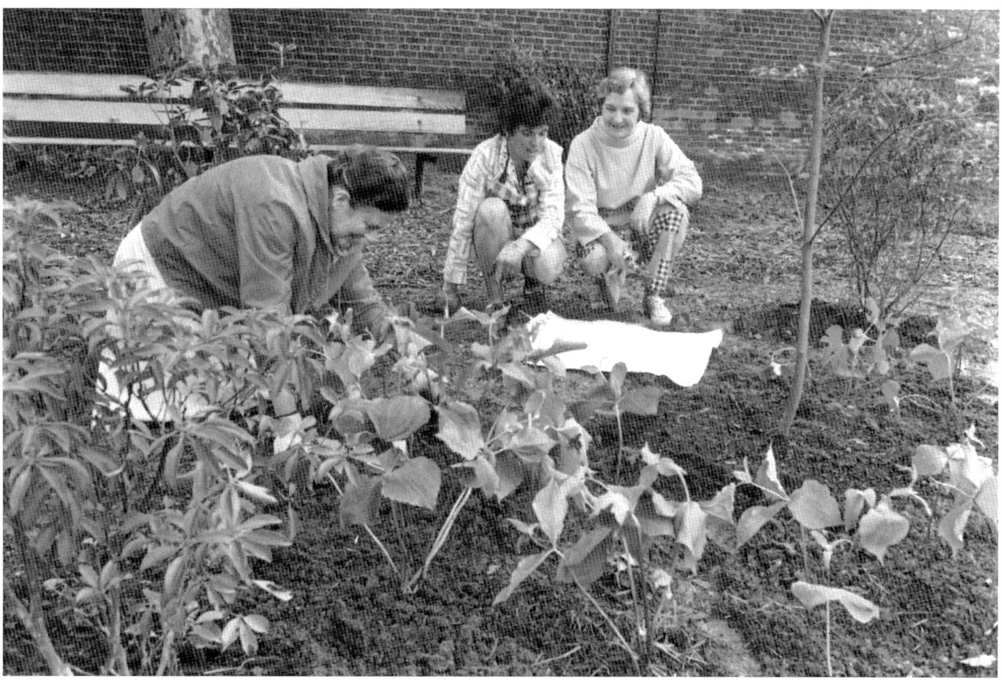

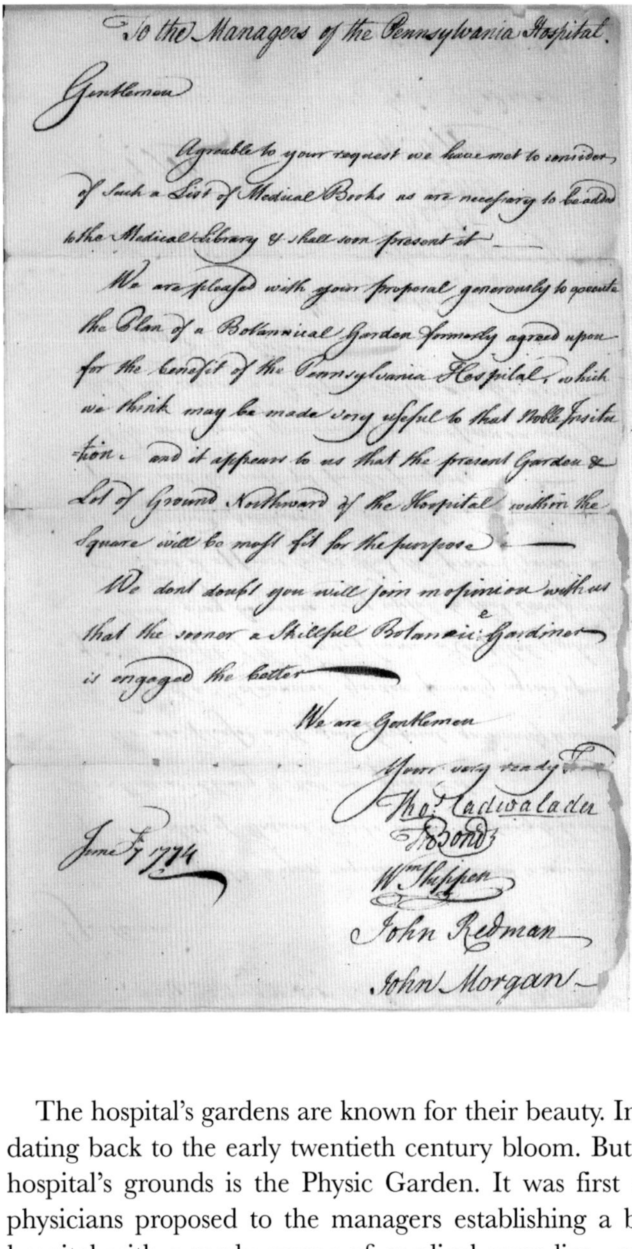

To the Managers of the Pennsylvania Hospital.

Gentlemen

Agreeable to your request we have met to consider of such a List of Medical Books as are necessary to be added to the Medical Library & shall soon present it —

We are pleased with your proposal generously to execute the Plan of a Botannical Garden formerly agreed upon for the benefit of the Pennsylvania Hospital, which we think may be made very useful to that Noble Institution. and it appears to us that the present Garden & Lot of Ground Northward of the Hospital within the Square will be most fit for the purpose —

We dont doubt you will join in opinion with us that the sooner a Skillful Botanic Gardiner is engaged the better —

We are Gentlemen

Your very ready [illegible]

Thos Cadwalader

Thos Bond

Wm Shippen

John Redman

John Morgan

June 7 1774

A June 7, 1774 letter to the board of managers, signed by the hospital physicians, asking for a gardener to be hired. They argued that hiring a gardener would reduce the cost of medicine by growing whatever herbs/plants they needed. *Courtesy of the Pennsylvania Hospital, Philadelphia, Administrative Records Collection.*

The hospital's gardens are known for their beauty. In the spring, wisteria and azaleas dating back to the early twentieth century bloom. But perhaps the crown jewel in the hospital's grounds is the Physic Garden. It was first mentioned in June 1774, when physicians proposed to the managers establishing a botanical garden to provide the hospital with a ready source of medical remedies—most medicines of the day were based on plant material. But the garden never materialized, mostly because of finances. However, in 1976, the Philadelphia Committee of the Garden Club of America and the Friends of Pennsylvania Hospital banded together to make the Physic Garden a reality.[135] The garden, with its foxglove (a plant whose leaves are used for making the medicine digitalis) and juniper (whose berries yield an ointment for wounds), is full of plants and herbs popular in the eighteenth century. It does not serve as early doctors thought it would, but instead serves to educate visitors.[136] Through the "Learn to Grow" program, begun in 2006, local schoolchildren are educated about the history of herbal medicine and its contributions to science and society.

THE CONTEMPORARY HOSPITAL, 1951–PRESENT

TWO CENTURIES OF CARE: THE FIRST FEMALE INTERN

In 1951, the hospital celebrated its 200th anniversary, marking 2.2 million patients treated since the days of Bond and Franklin. It was also in that year that the first female intern was admitted. Nancy George Boucot, a native Philadelphian and graduate of the University of Pennsylvania's School of Medicine, was recommended for her high marks and for being a "pleasant gentlewoman."[137] After her successful year-long internship, hospital administrator John Hatfield wrote that "although Pennsylvania Hospital has been in existence 200 years, Doctor Boucot is the first woman intern we have had here. In no way have we regretted the appointment."[138]

THE CATHCART ERA BRINGS MODERNIZATION, SPECIALTIES

In 1949, H. Robert Cathcart was hired as assistant hospital administrator. The Cathcart era at the hospital would continue for forty-two years—he was promoted to administrator in 1952 and elevated to president in 1970, a position he held until he retired in 1991. When the twenty-four-year-old Iowan arrived at Pennsylvania Hospital, he recalls, "It was a quality medical establishment who had a very good board and a very good history of caring for the sick poor." That focus on the indigent came at the expense of the hospital's physical plant, though. When Cathcart's tenure began, patients still stayed in forty-bed and twenty-two-bed wards, with very few private rooms. The hospital was meticulously kept, but it ran on direct current it generated itself; most private rooms did not have plumbing and certainly no modern conveniences such as call buttons. While other hospitals in the city had moved away from the ward model, Pennsylvania Hospital's physical plant was decidedly antiquated.

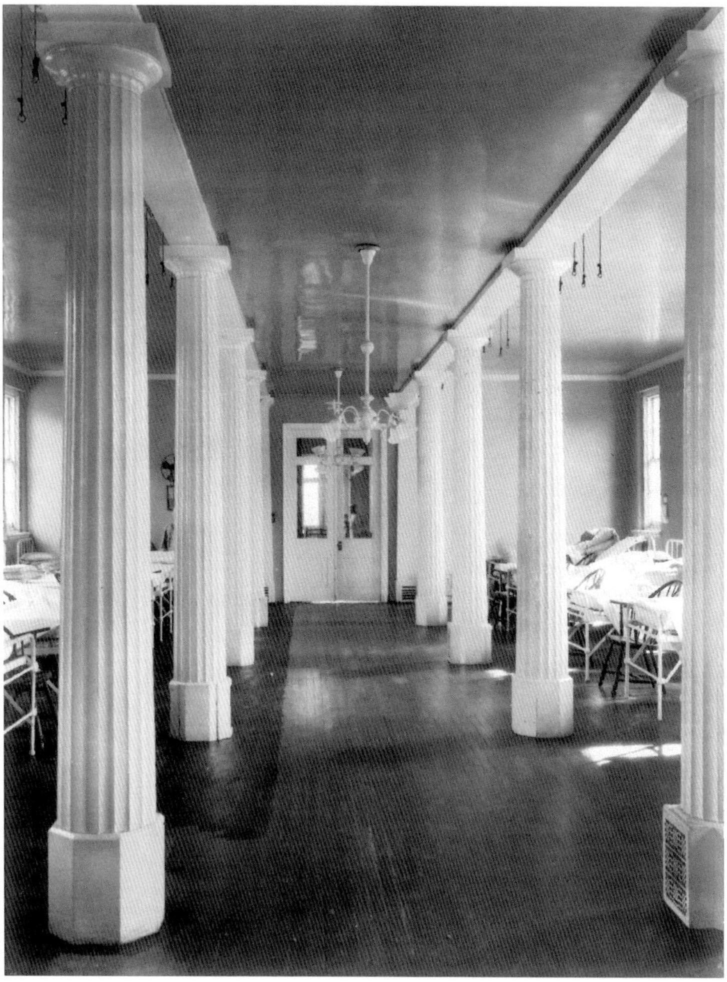

An early twentieth-century image of the Medical Ward, East Wing of the Pine Building. Patient beds line the ward. *Courtesy of the Pennsylvania Hospital, Philadelphia, PAH Image Collection 769c.*

Though the hospital offered excellent care, it had few specialists. Still, it "was a coveted place for interns. They came here with no salary, room and board only, and laundry. The residents in medicine started out at twenty dollars a month and each year went up ten dollars a month," Cathcart remembers.[139]

Dr. Robert Gill arrived as an intern in 1948, one of the last crop of two-year interns. (He would stay at the hospital through 1998.) In those days, intern candidates submitted to interviews by the board of managers. "We sat on an old Quaker bench outside the big room, sweating and waiting," he said.[140] Once inside, the board—businessmen and lawyers, experienced in hiring and firing—grilled the would-be interns on their interests, schooling and the nature of their characters. The interns were a close-knit group who lived in the Pine Building, using the Historic Surgical Amphitheatre as their lounge. "We had a TV set in there, and we'd sit around and talk. Every Friday night, a cookie jar would appear, put there by the hospital. It was supposed to be Ben Franklin's cookie jar." A large, leather-bound book dating back to the nineteenth century sat on a table for the interns to use and often to pore over. "People would write in it—interesting things they saw in their work. It had a lot of marvelous stuff in it. It was a marvelous archive."[141] From internships onward, the doctors were encouraged to think of the sick poor. The noted Dr. Garfield Duncan told his doctors that if they wanted to admit patients, they had to work in clinics for the poor, Gill remembers. He did so until he was sixty-six years old. "It was a good way—it gave people who couldn't afford it the chance to see chiefs as well as interns and residents."[142]

Under Cathcart's watch, the hospital began to boom in the 1950s and 1960s, turning into a modern acute care institution and adding expertise in several specialties. An intensive care unit for neurological patients, a coronary care unit, an orthopedic institute, a diabetes center, a hospice, specialized units in oncology and urology and broadened surgical programs all blossomed. Dr. Terrence Malloy, now chief of urology at the hospital, was recruited by Cathcart. He started at the hospital in August 1968, the first of a string of doctors who would build Pennsylvania Hospital into a modern tertiary care facility. "Mr. Cathcart was trying to reestablish us as the preeminent hospital of Philadelphia, just as it was in the early days," Dr. Malloy said.[143]

Attracting young, talented physicians was a winning strategy. "Pennsylvania Hospital really promoted the young physicians and allowed them to become preeminent in their field," said Dr. Malloy.[144] Some of the advances were able to happen because of a series of grants given by the Hartford Foundation, a New York nonprofit that awarded the hospital a dozen separate awards in all, some of which attracted top specialists to set up shop at Pennsylvania Hospital.[145]

During these years, private patients—attracting them and caring for them—became emphasized in a way they had not been before, and much of that had to do with a growing healthcare phenomenon, a new insurance company called Blue Cross. "We recognized that this newfangled Blue Cross was going to start paying for people, and we had to take advantage of that," Cathcart said.

The challenge was not to abandon the charge to care for the sick poor, but to also care for other patients who would help subsidize those whom Dr. Bond and Franklin envisioned as Pennsylvania Hospital's core consumer.[146] Cathcart also convinced the board of the need to build modern facilities. He oversaw the renovation of some structures and the construction of new ones to meet the demand for privacy. Still, Cathcart and his board were careful to keep the spirit of Franklin and Dr. Bond alive, opening clinics and community health centers.[147]

As the hospital was building and growing, a group of ex-residents devoted to the hospital's history shone a light on Jacob Ehrenzeller, the hospital's first resident. "As you stayed here, you got very appreciative of the history. It really got into you," said Dr. Gill. In the 1960s, Dr. Gill began researching Ehrenzeller, even contacting the Chester County Historical Society to find out as much as he could about the man. The historical society had happened upon a portrait of Ehrenzeller in an antique shop. It purchased the work, and Dr. Gill decided the hospital should have a copy of the portrait. With Cathcart's blessing, Dr. Gill reached out to all of the hospital's ex-residents around the world and asked them to contribute to a fund to commission the work. "The money kept pouring in," Dr. Gill remembers. "It was such a loyal group." Once the artwork was complete, the annual Jacob Ehrenzeller Award for service in medicine was conceived and given, first to Dr. Francis Lukens, a national figure in diabetes who had done his internship and residency at Pennsylvania Hospital.[148]

Many attributed this time of growth and specialization to Cathcart, a strong leader who made the hospital his home. He lived across the street, and he or his wife, Tressa, could often be found patrolling the halls at odd hours, talking to patients and staff. He rode through the neighborhood on his bicycle. "He was very much a hands-on guy, and a huge influence on the hospital, on its progress," said Morris Cheston Jr., the chairman of the board of managers, a man whose father held the same position and whose own affiliation with the hospital dates back to the 1980s.[149] Cathcart's influence extended beyond the hospital. He served as president and chairman of the Delaware Valley Hospital Council, the Hospital Association of Pennsylvania and the American Hospital Association. When he retired in 1991, Pennsylvania Hospital renamed its Core Building in his honor.[150]

Early Merger Talks: Changes in Healthcare, a New Partnership

Over time, the campuses of Pennsylvania Hospital and Thomas Jefferson University grew until they nearly met. By 1973, at Tenth and Spruce, Pennsylvania Hospital began one block east and Jefferson was less than a block north. Each hospital had something to gain from the other—Jefferson regarded Pennsylvania Hospital's psychiatric services as a boon, and Pennsylvania Hospital looked to improve its maternity services with an affiliation with Jefferson. The two announced they were weighing a merger in March 1973. Talks were broken off quickly, however; hospital officials cited possible interference with Pennsylvania Hospital programs and a strong desire to continue partnering with the University of Pennsylvania's School of Medicine.[151] During his tenure, Cathcart said, affiliating with Jefferson was weighed three separate times, with varying degrees of seriousness.[152]

The shifting dynamics of the healthcare reimbursement landscape began to affect Pennsylvania Hospital dramatically in the 1980s. The traditional cost-based system was changing to a prospective pricing system, and it meant big changes for hospitals nationally. Pressure mounted to keep costs down, shorten stays and perform outpatient procedures whenever possible. The challenge for Pennsylvania Hospital, and all hospitals, was to keep patient care high while maintaining the bottom line.[153] It was a challenge that would become increasingly difficult as the years went by.

Pressures to cut costs and deal with healthcare reform caused the hospital to partner with Thomas Jefferson University in 1993. The alliance was not a merger, but a deal to share resources, eliminate duplication of services and consolidate medical leadership. It was the most significant alliance Pennsylvania Hospital made up until that time, and it came against a backdrop of hospital mergers, consolidations and affiliations regionally and nationwide. Costs were rising, revenue was stagnating, government subsidies were being cut and a new managed-care philosophy of health insurance coverage and reduced Medicare reimbursement were all issues to contend with. Hospital networks were a response to declining occupancy and pressures from insurance companies to slash spending. In a short time, however, it became clear that the alliance did not do enough to position Pennsylvania Hospital. In 1992, the hospital reported $10 million profit. In 1996, it didn't break even.[154]

A CROSSROADS: THE FUTURE OF THE INSTITUTE

The crossroads at which the hospital found itself in the late 1990s forced the board of managers into making difficult choices. One of these tough issues was the future of the Institute of Pennsylvania Hospital. Once a pioneer in the field and a national model for mental health treatment, it was now a financial drain on the hospital. In 1992, the Institute posted a profit of $2.8 million. But in the subsequent four years, its losses mounted, including a $2 million deficit in 1995 and a $4 million deficit in 1996.[155] Those losses snowballed to the point that the Institute was losing $1.5 million a month, according to then-president and CEO Dr. John R. Ball.[156]

Patient stays were declining, too—from an average of nearly forty days in 1992 to about eight days in 1997, a shift that meant less reimbursement and revenue for the Institute. Long-term, intensive, personalized care had been a hallmark of the Institute since the days of Thomas Story Kirkbride. But in the 1990s, with insurers less willing to pay for extended care, lengthy stays by and large became a thing of the past. Treatment was increasingly shifting to community mental health facilities, with patients either choosing or being forced into these options rather than hospitalization. The patient census dropped from perhaps 200 at any given time in the mid-1980s to about 115 in 1996.

On October 12, 1996, the board announced it was selling the Institute and the twenty-seven-acre site it had occupied since 1840. CoreCare Systems Inc., a private firm set up in 1994 to own and manage psychiatric care facilities, purchased the Institute for $4.5 million.[157] In the final weeks of Pennsylvania Hospital ownership, the center had only about a dozen patients. The sale was finalized in February 1997. CoreCare's plans included subdividing the site into parcels that would make up a campus of different types of medical care facilities, including a nursing home, assisted-living residences, offices for private psychiatric patients, an adult day-care center, a home-healthcare facility and retail stores. Pennsylvania Hospital, meanwhile, transferred 66 of its remaining 195 employees to the Eighth and Spruce site, and planned to maintain twenty-four beds for psychiatric care there, as compared to more than two hundred at the Institute.[158]

The years after the separation proved unsteady for the former Institute, now renamed the Kirkbride Center by CoreCare and reinvented as a 120-bed facility. In

2005, CoreCare leased campus space to organizations such as the West Philadelphia Charter School, Baptist Children's Services, Early Head Start program and the Mill Creek School, the high school for troubled teenagers that continues to be operated by Pennsylvania Hospital.[159]

THE FUTURE OF THE HOSPITAL

Losses at the Institute were a single symptom of a larger problem. The declining ability of the hospital to maintain financial viability itself was a huge question that the board needed to address. Marketplace forces were causing hospitals around the country to merge or affiliate to join resources, achieve economies of scale and, especially crucial in the waning days of the twentieth century, gain added clout in bargaining with healthcare insurers for bigger payments.

There was a fundamental shift in the economics of healthcare—traditional fee-for-service arrangements meant that hospitals with the most patients and most services had the most revenue. But in a managed-care environment, hospitals that fare best financially are those that can keep patients out of expensive hospital beds and in primary or outpatient facilities.[160] Moreover, in a marketplace where healthcare consumers have multiple choices, the cachet of a big-name institution was also a factor to consider. Pennsylvania Hospital earned $10 million in profit in 1992, but by 1996 it lost $3 million. The number of patients covered by managed care doubled from 20 percent to 40 percent in the same period, meaning that the hospital was coping with a great percentage of minimal payments for services and procedures.[161] These rapid changes were happening everywhere. "It has moved from a strong institution, a pillar in the community, to an endangered species," a healthcare consultant told a *Philadelphia Inquirer* reporter. "You can be threatened and gone in essentially the blink of an eye."[162]

Losing the independence that had been a hallmark of the institution since 1751 was a very real possibility, and in 1995 the board began studying whether to affiliate with the Jefferson Health System or the University of Pennsylvania Health System (UPHS). It was a painful decision, but a necessary one. "We literally had to make sure the hospital survived by joining a health system," said Dr. Michael Buckley, chief medical officer of the hospital, who was heavily involved in the merger.[163] Pennsylvania Hospital had longstanding academic and other ties to both potential partners. The connection to Penn was a historic one—hospital co-founder Benjamin Franklin had also founded the University of Pennsylvania, and the hospital had served as a training ground for Penn medical students since the eighteenth century.[164]

Board members weighed the business strength of UPHS against what was perceived as the potential for greater autonomy under a Jefferson alliance. October 28, 1996, was supposed to be the date of a decisive meeting on the issue, but the members remained split and postponed a decision until more information could be gathered. Professional staff members were about equally split on the question, as well. Two weeks later, on

November 12, managers again met in a special session. They were initially still divided, but cast several secret ballots until they arrived at consensus on affiliating with UPHS, which operated the Hospital of the University of Pennsylvania, Presbyterian Medical Center and Phoenixville Hospital.

The Jefferson system reacted swiftly, pledging to compete head-on with its former partner. Some Pennsylvania Hospital doctors had previously held faculty appointments at Jefferson Medical College, so those physicians had to choose whether to retain those ties.[165] One reason the board favored Penn was the physical proximity of Jefferson to Pennsylvania Hospital—Jefferson was just a few blocks away from the hospital. Some believed that had the board chosen Jefferson, Jefferson would have closed all or part of Pennsylvania Hospital because the two were serving essentially the same areas of Society Hill, South Philadelphia and Camden, New Jersey. Penn is located in West Philadelphia and represented less of an overlap of service area.

At the time, hospital president John Ball characterized the combination as Pennsylvania Hospital becoming a subsidiary of UPHS, retaining its name, identity and local governance, while still reporting and being accountable to Penn. Even with the tough choice finally made, Moody's Investors service lowered the hospital's bond rating and criticized the board's "history of indecision" on the question. It cast doubt on the Penn affiliation and cited the potential for many defections of Pennsylvania Hospital doctors, and their patient bases, to Jefferson.[166] Originally, UPHS and Pennsylvania Hospital had discussed a two- to five-year transition period, but by May 1997, "market conditions"—in part the withdrawal of doctors—forced the negotiators to accelerate the timetable by about two years.[167] The combination of the two entities became effective on October 31, 1997, and the independent board of managers ceased to exist. Under a post-merger agreement, UPHS appoints two-thirds of the managers, the chair is independent, another member is independent and one seat is occupied by a Pennsylvania Hospital physician. The board no longer crafts the hospital's budget or wields decision-making authority; it is largely an information-sharing body. The money that UPHS paid to acquire Pennsylvania Hospital was used to create and fund a foundation, the First Hospital Foundation.

The predicted loss of doctors to Jefferson did take place after the merger, and a corresponding drop in revenue also happened. Things went from bad to worse, financially. The hospital ended 1998 with a $30 million deficit. As a result, officials closed two floors of patient-care facilities—the seventh floor of the Scheidt Building and the seventh floor of the Cathcart Building.[168] The system at large also experienced financial woes. Its worst-ever financial performance happened in 1998, with a $90 million loss and a projected $150 million loss for the following fiscal year.[169] Instead, it turned out to be even worse, with UPHS posting a $198 million loss that year.[170] "I think there is a serious crisis in American medicine at the moment," UPHS system chief executive Dr. William N. Kelley said at the time, pointing to cutbacks in Medicare reimbursement, reduced and delayed payments from insurers and rising numbers of uninsured and underinsured patients.[171]

The health system laid off eleven hundred employees two months later and hired the Hunter Group, a Florida-based healthcare consulting firm with a reputation for turning around struggling organizations by implementing aggressive cost-cutting and restructuring measures.[172] That October, UPHS announced seventeen hundred more layoffs. In all, there were three separate layoffs within eighteen months. The effect at Pennsylvania Hospital was pronounced—it lost nine hundred of its three thousand positions, and those who remained were asked to do more work. At times, said Morris Cheston Jr., chairman of the board of managers, things looked even darker than before the merger—the financially troubled health system explored the possibility of either closing or selling Pennsylvania Hospital. "It was a very big issue for a while," Cheston said.[173]

In the face of all the cuts, Tim Morgan, then–executive director of the hospital, promised that patients would not see a difference in bedside care, a view that some doctors and staff disputed, but that the hospital would focus on five areas of specialization: orthopedics, women's health, cardiology, cancer treatment and neurosciences.[174] Among those who were laid off were longtime employees with twenty-five to thirty years of service to the hospital. Those who remained at the hospital were left with heavier workloads, and morale suffered. "It was very rocky initially," said Kathleen Kinslow, the hospital's executive director. "I think the same things would have happened if we had joined with Jefferson, but people blamed the decision that was made, said we should have stayed freestanding. It's taken us almost a decade to heal from that."[175]

EMERGING FROM A DIFFICULT TIME

Despite the pain, a new focus brought results. The hospital pared down to its core specialties—"babies, bones, and brains," as Kinslow puts it, or maternity care, including high-risk obstetrics and fertility; orthopedics, including joint replacement techniques; and the neurosciences. They are the areas for which Pennsylvania Hospital is known and the areas with a high volume of patient care. And it rededicated itself to its people, building consensus among physicians, staff and patients. The health system emerged from its financial troubles, and the hospital found its place in the larger system.

With the power of the University of Pennsylvania Health System behind it, the hospital was able to do some things more effectively, including collecting payments and getting better reimbursement from third-party payers. "We're a much bigger player—we're Penn, we're Presby, we're Pennsylvania Hospital, we're the major player in town. We can negotiate much better deals," said Cheston.[176] Hard work has yielded results—after the painful rebuilding period, the hospital again earns profits annually.[177] And though some feared becoming part of the University of Pennsylvania Health System would mean the hospital would lose its identity, that has not been the case. "The system has its own identity, and each of the entities has their own identity," said Kinslow. "There is a real feeling of respect for what Pennsylvania Hospital is and there is an intense desire for us to maintain who we are."[178]

THE CONTEMPORARY HOSPITAL: LOOKING AHEAD

A focus on patient care continues to be a hallmark of the contemporary Pennsylvania Hospital. The hospital is staffed by physicians who want to practice almost exclusively clinical medicine, as opposed to research. These doctors want to teach, and they bring a very high academic sensibility to the hospital. "It makes for a focus on patient care, but a very high quality, and a focus on teaching the next generation," says Dr. Michael Buckley. "It's a very high quality staff."

Chief of urology Dr. Terrence Malloy puts it this way: "The hospital supports the physicians in what they want to do, and that doesn't often happen. Here, they see that it is the unique physician that's going to draw patients to a Center City hospital, away from suburban hospitals and New Jersey hospitals."[179]

As it moves forward, the hospital faces multiple challenges, as all modern healthcare organizations do. Chief among them is the malpractice crisis—insurance premiums for healthcare providers are skyrocketing, making it difficult for some physicians to do business at all. A tough labor market is also an issue—shortages in nurses, physical therapists and radiologists. "You want to make sure that you have the right labor force that is competent and will provide high-quality care to your patients, but it's a competitive marketplace right now," Kinslow says. "I believe it will continue to be that way well into the future." In the wake of fourteen local hospitals shutting down their maternity units in the past decade, more babies than ever are born at Pennsylvania Hospital, with 4,839 deliveries in 2006. It is a delicate balance to negotiate growing a department and its infrastructure needs with very limited operating margins.

The economic reality is that obstetric care is expensive, and reimbursements from insurance companies are low; the malpractice crisis is especially acute in the area of obstetrics.[180] Experts worry about capital dollars—how to keep enough cash on hand to buy the latest equipment needed to compete for and serve today's sophisticated healthcare consumers. For-profit healthcare providers can borrow money, but nonprofits such as Pennsylvania Hospital are limited in the ways they can raise funds.[181]

Pennsylvania Hospital's Center City location presents its own set of issues. "There are increasing challenges for hospitals who are in inner cities in terms of uninsured and underinsured people. We don't turn them away, and that's a financial challenge," said Dr. Buckley.[182] Also, regulatory issues and increased reporting demands are a drain on resources. People who were once at bedsides are now needed to record data by hand. "I believe in transparency; it's important that the public can make informed decisions, but information technology hasn't yet caught up," Kinslow says. Patients are also coming to the hospital with greater acuity, but their lengths of stay are shorter. Rather than looking at care in episodic bursts, "we need to look at a continuum of care to be on the forefront. That's how Pennsylvania Hospital will maintain the niche that it has in the marketplace."[183]

Another concern moving forward will be preserving the historic Pine Building, which, buffeted by 250-plus years of wind and rain, needs millions of dollars of costly repairs.

In 2006, the hospital launched a $7 million campaign to perform necessary repairs and to build an endowment dedicated to the upkeep of the eighteenth-century edifice. Now, with scarce capital dollars, "we decide, do we put a new roof on the Pine Building, or do we buy ten more respirators for infants. The answer is always ten more respirators for infants. We don't want to have to make those decisions; there should be a fund so there's enough for both. It's very important to the staff and the community to preserve this historic place," said Dr. Michael Buckley, the hospital's chief medical officer.[184]

Moving forward, the hospital looks to position itself as a destination hospital. It will not be able to survive as only a community-based facility; it must continue to attract and retain top-notch physicians, keep up with technology and build on its well-known, high-end services such as neurology, obstetrics, cardiology, orthopedics, psychiatry and cancer to draw patients from far away.[185]

PAST AND FUTURE

Pennsylvania Hospital has survived for more than 250 years, not because it has stayed the same, but because it has changed appropriately with the times.

Still, a sense of history permeates the place. It even looks different from its peers. "When you go to other hospitals, they all look the same. We look different. When I first arrived here, I fell in love with the place," Dr. Buckley said. For as long as it has existed, there has been a real sense of community at America's first hospital. History still matters. A case in point: in 2007, the hospital began the process of refining its vision statement, setting out with the goals of something forward-looking and cutting-edge. But person after person kept coming back and saying that no articulation of the hospital's vision could be complete without a nod to its rich past.

It's a good bet that should Dr. Bond and Benjamin Franklin stroll today into the hospital they founded, they would be quite satisfied. "They would be proud," said Dr. Buckley. "They would be very happy to see the Pine building still here and in good shape. I think they would be very happy to see that it's a thriving enterprise and that we still care for the sick poor, for the mentally ill. I think they would be pleased with what we've done with their hospital."[186]

Dr. Malloy agrees. "It's a hospital with a historic name, and it came back to be a powerful force in the new millennium."[187]

PENNSYLVANIA HOSPITAL: A TIMELINE

1751, January 23	"Sundry inhabitants of the said Province" present a petition to the Provincial Assembly of Pennsylvania seeking authority to establish a hospital for the poor, sick, injured and "distemper'd in Mind and Deprived of their rational Faculties."
1751, May 11	Provincial Assembly issues a charter for Pennsylvania Hospital, which is approved by Lieutenant Governor James Hamilton.
1751, July 1	First meeting of contributors to the hospital is held in the statehouse; they elect twelve managers and a treasurer to govern the hospital's operation.
1751, July 6	Managers meet and elect Joshua Crosby as president and Benjamin Franklin as clerk.
1751, July	Managers appoint Franklin and Thomas Bond to design a corporate seal.
1751, September 2	First donation of real estate for the benefit of the hospital, by Mathias Kaplan.
1751, October 23	First medical staff is appointed.
1751, November 28	First matron, Elizabeth Gardner, is appointed to oversee housekeeping and general patient care.
1752, February 10	Hospital opened in temporary quarters, in Judge John Kinsey's mansion on Market Street (south side of Market Street, then called High Street, below Seventh Street.) The board meets to consider applications from prospective patients.
1752, February 11	The first patient, Margaret Sherlock, is admitted.
1752, March 5	First paying psychiatric patient, a female, is admitted.
1752, December 7	Hospital's apothecary shop is opened, and Jonathan Roberts is appointed as the first apothecary upon the recommendation of Dr. Thomas Bond.
1752, December 13	First outpatient service, then called dispensary, is opened. First patient reportedly was treated for a case of "periodic madness."
1754, February	The hospital seal, bearing the image of the Good Samaritan, is completed.

1754, May 28	Franklin presents his manuscript, *Some Account of the Pennsylvania Hospital from its First Beginning to the Fifth Month, Called May, 1754.* The board of managers orders fifteen hundred copies published.
1754, September 11	Board purchases ground for permanent hospital, facing Pine Street, for £500.
1755	Wounded and ill soldiers from the French and Indian War are treated at the hospital.
1755, May 28	Cornerstone is laid in ceremonies, with Benjamin Franklin in attendance.
1755, June 30	Franklin is elected second president of the board of managers; he serves until 1757, when he left to serve as provincial agent in England.
1755, December 27	First meeting of the board of managers in the nearly completed Pine Street building is held.
1756, May 6	First meeting of contributors in new Pine Street permanent facility is held.
1756, December 17	Patients in the temporary hospital on Market Street are moved to the new hospital, the East Wing of the Pine Street structure.
1759, December 28	Theatrical production of Shakespeare's *Hamlet* is held as a benefit for the hospital.
1762, July 27	Board of managers receives a gift of a medical book from Dr. John Fothergill of London, the first book in what would become the hospital's medical library.
1763	Dr. William Shippen Jr. begins first medical lectures at the hospital.
1765	The first medical school in the country is founded by Dr. John Morgan and Dr. William Shippen Jr. at the College of Philadelphia, later the University of Pennsylvania. Pennsylvania Hospital's affiliation with the medical school continues today.
1765, July 17	First child is born at Pennsylvania Hospital, the "female child of Martha Robinson, a poor patient."
1765	First gallstone operation in the country is performed at the hospital.
1766	Dr. Thomas Bond institutes the first course of medical instruction for America's first medical students.
1767, November 10	Richard and Thomas Penn, proprietors of the Province of Pennsylvania, donate a strip of ground, giving the board of managers control of all the property between Eighth and Ninth Streets between Pine and Spruce Streets, about 4.3 acres in all.
1773	Jacob Ehrenzeller, the first medical resident, is appointed, and serves for five years.

1776	During the American Revolution, the hospital cares for both British and Continental soldiers. It endures the exile of four members of the board of managers, and it suffers financially for years to come. Dr. Benjamin Rush, later a staff member, writes a definitive treatise on military medicine that serves the nation until the Civil War.
1777	British occupy the Pennsylvania Hospital, affecting the care of the patients.
1778, June 17	British occupation of the hospital, and Philadelphia, ends.
1780	The board of managers, concerned about fire prevention given the hospital's use of candles for light and fireplaces for heating, purchases an early American hand-pumper fire engine. Proud of their purchase, the board declares that "the fire engine [shall be] played every month at the meetings of the board." The engine remains at the hospital today.
1786	The Philadelphia Dispensary is opened. This outpatient service, which in 1800 was located at Fifth and Chestnut, affiliated with Pennsylvania Hospital in 1927.
1793	An epidemic of yellow fever hits Philadelphia from July to November, causing four thousand deaths; the board of managers suspends meetings. Approximately 10 percent of the city's population dies in the epidemic.
1794	Dr. Phillip Syng Physick is appointed to the staff; he will serve until 1816. He achieves fame through his surgical prowess and becomes known as the "father of American surgery."
1796	Construction of the second wing of the hospital, the West Wing, is completed; psychiatric patients are moved in under the care of Dr. Benjamin Rush, social reformer and signer of the Declaration of Independence. Center structure of Pine Building is completed; apothecary shop moves into the south room opposite the administration office.
1800, September	Artist Benjamin West is requested by the managers to create and donate a painting to the hospital.
1803, February	Lying-in (maternity) ward is opened on second floor, East Wing, of the Pine Building.
1804	Managers order the maintenance of systematic medical histories with a record book of each case treated at the hospital. The book was laid out at every monthly meeting.
1804	Surgical amphitheatre is opened in the new center portion of the Pine Building, which joins the previously separate East and West Wings. The amphitheatre, the first of its kind, featured space for students and observers, and was used until 1868.
1804, September 24	Cast-lead statue of William Penn arrives from London on the ship *Pigou*. The statue is donated to the hospital by John Penn, William Penn's grandson.

1805	Managers invite Dr. Philip Syng Physick to occupy the first "chair of surgery."
1807	First City Troop of Cavalry donates the entire sum of their pay from the Revolutionary War, received many years late, to the Lying-in Department. This endowment is given to be used "in such a manner and proportion as the Managers think proper."
1807, October 26	Historical medical library first occupies its quarters on the second story of the Pine Building.
1808	Ten years after Edward Jenner publishes his findings that vaccinating with cowpox prevents smallpox, the board of managers advertises in local newspapers that the "Poor of Pennsylvania shall be vaccinated gratis, if they will call at the Hospital."
1811	The first American anatomy textbook is published by Dr. Caspar Wistar, a renowned teacher who joined the hospital's medical staff in 1793.
1812	The first psychiatric textbook in America is published by Dr. Benjamin Rush.
1817, October	Benjamin West's oil painting *Christ Healing the Sick in the Temple* arrives at the hospital.
1818	West Picture House is constructed to house and display the West painting. In the first twelve months that the canvas is on display, thirty thousand visitors come to see it, and the hospital raises $15,000 by charging admission.
1830	Lying-in department is closed for the first time due to an outbreak of puerperal fever.
1831, November 18	U.S. Chief Justice John Marshall presents a gift of a silver wine cooler to Dr. Philip Syng Physick in appreciation for a successful operation.
1832	A resolution is passed: "Resolved…a separate Asylum be provided for our insane patients with ample space for their proper seclusion, classification and employment."
1835	During the mild winter, the hospital earns revenue by selling ice—probably cut from ponds at Third and Pine and Ninth and South—stored in two hospital icehouses built in 1794 and 1811.
1836, February	Managers name a committee to pursue construction on newly purchased land in West Philadelphia.
1836, June 22	Cornerstone is laid at Forty-fourth Street Psychiatric Department in West Philadelphia.
1840, October 12	Dr. Thomas Story Kirkbride becomes the physician in chief of the psychiatric hospital.

1841, January 1	The building in West Philadelphia is opened for psychiatric patients. It later becomes the Institute of Pennsylvania Hospital. Dr. Thomas Story Kirkbride becomes the superintendent of the new Department for the Insane and moves to the new grounds with his family, spending the rest of his life devoted to the creation of a humane world for the mentally ill.
1844, October 15	American Psychiatric Association, then called the Association of Medical Superintendents of American Institutions for the Insane, is founded at a meeting of Dr. Kirkbride and twelve other administrators, held at the West Philadelphia psychiatric department.
1846–1847	Anesthesia is introduced at the hospital. No written record of the date of its introduction exists, but Dr. James Darrach, who was on staff during these years, related that while at the hospital, Dr. George Norris, the surgeon on duty, ordered him to get some ether and try it on a patient.
1847	The American Medical Association designates Pennsylvania Hospital's Medical Library as the first, as well as the largest and most important, in the United States.
1851	At the direction of the board of managers, Dr. George B. Wood prepares a history of the first century of the hospital.
1851, January 27	Main entrance is moved from Pine Street to Eighth Street. Lying-in Department (maternity) is disbanded. It cost nearly $20,000 in excess of the endowment, principal and interest, from the City Troop fund.
1856, July 9	Construction begins on West Philadelphia psychiatric facility for men. Then known as the Department for Insane Men, the building became known as "Kirkbride's Hospital."
1856, October 1	Cornerstone is laid for Kirkbride's Hospital.
1859	Five blocks west of the Pennsylvania Hospital for the Insane, a twin version of the mental hospital is opened at Forty-ninth and Market Streets. The original campus becomes the Department for Females, and the newer campus is the Department for Males.
1861	Pennsylvania Hospital's surgical expertise brings 124 casualties to its wards for special treatment during the Civil War. As in the American Revolution, the hospital experiences the severe economic consequences of war; most of the city's leading charitable institutions are inadequately funded.
1865, February	Board of managers appoints a Committee of Women Visitors to promote the "mental, moral, and spiritual welfare of the patients."
1866, May 7	At the annual contributors' meeting, the first suggestion of a nursing school is made.

1875, December 27	Board of managers appoints Dr. J. Forsyth Meigs, an attending physician and former resident physician at the hospital, to write a history of the hospital covering the period from its centennial in 1851 to 1876.
1875	The hospital's first training program for nurses is proposed and developed. A formal one-year course of instruction is offered and includes students from the Women's Hospital of Philadelphia from 1879 to 1882. In 1883, an independent school is established and the first class of four students is graduated in 1884. Three 1885 graduates achieved a first—they are assigned to the Men's Medical Ward. Because of the outstanding work of these three, hereafter trained women nurses are employed on all medical wards, male and female.
1876	Hospital purchases Philadelphia's first known ambulance, a horse-drawn vehicle that resembled a bread wagon. The ambulance, harness, et cetera, cost $400. A horse was donated to the hospital.
1876, September 25	Dr. J. Forsyth Meigs reads his address, *A History of the First Quarter of the Second Century of the Pennsylvania Hospital*, at a board of managers meeting; the manuscript is published in book form the following year.
1886, March 1	Three female nurses are placed in a male ward for the first time.
1887, April 23	The first planned appendectomy is performed at the hospital by Dr. Thomas G. Morton.
1892, May	Construction begins on the nurses' home.
1893, February 27	Nurses' home is opened and furnished at Ninth and Spruce Streets.
1895	Dr. Thomas G. Morton publishes his *History of Pennsylvania Hospital 1751–1895.*
1895, October 28	Lucy Walker is appointed superintendent of nursing at the Eighth Street site.
1897	Hospital purchases its first X-ray machine, two years after Wilhelm Roentgen's description of X-rays shocked and amazed the Western world.
1897, April 23	Walter Garrett Memorial Building is opened at Eighth and Spruce Streets, on the site of the former "Elaboratory."
1898	Josephine Mellon Ayer bequeaths $50,000 to the hospital to establish the Ayer Clinical Laboratory. A subsequent gift by her son, Frederick Fanning Ayer, in his mother's memory, allowed for the publication of bulletins of the laboratory's work.
1898	Close to three hundred soldiers are admitted to the hospital, after being wounded in the Spanish-American War. Some of them are transported from distant ports of entry on special Red Cross trains manned by Pennsylvania Hospital staff.

1912	Hospital replaces horse-drawn ambulance service with automobile ambulance service. The original ambulance driver, Dick Howard, who had held the ambulance driver job for almost thirty years, was so attached to the horse that when he got word the hospital would be switching to a gasoline-powered ambulance, he collapsed. "I drove the new motor ambulance for a few months, but it wasn't for me. There wasn't the thrill there was in driving a horse," he told a newspaper reporter in 1931.
1914	Pennsylvania Hospital School of Nursing for Men is opened, providing training for male nurses in the areas of behavioral health and genitourinary tract therapies. It is the first training school for male nurses in the United States to be headed by a man, Leroy N. Craig.
1917, May 18	Pennsylvania Hospital Unit Base No. 10, sets sail for France in World War I. The hospital is at the forefront of hospital service units, and it lasts for twenty-one months in France. Almost ten thousand patients are treated.
1919, January 14	Name of Pennsylvania Hospital for the Insane, Forty-ninth and Market Streets, is changed to Pennsylvania Hospital Department for Medical and Nervous Diseases.
1926	Pennsylvania Lying-in Hospital affiliates with Pennsylvania Hospital, the first step toward a merger.
1926, May	Construction begins on outpatient building, Eighth and Spruce Streets.
1927	First electrocardiogram machine (ECG) is purchased. By now, patient records are standardized, typed and often contain pictures and graphs.
1927, December 6	Outpatient building on Spruce Street is opened, hospital's outpatient department affiliates with the historic Philadelphia Dispensary.
1928, September 17	Ground is broken on a $1.5 million building at Forty-ninth and Market.
1929, June 27	After a seventy-five-year hiatus, Pennsylvania Hospital reinstates obstetrics and gynecology with the Women's Building, now known as the Spruce Building. With 150 adult beds, eighty bassinets, two operating rooms and a series of labor and delivery rooms, as well as outpatient clinics, it is considered "one of the most modern hospital buildings in the country" and is so designated, well into the 1950s.
1930, March 1	Institute of the Pennsylvania Hospital is opened at Forty-ninth and Market Streets.
1933, April 18	Original Benjamin Franklin manuscript containing the inscription that was placed on the hospital's cornerstone is sold to the hospital at cost by an antique dealer who found it in Germany.

1938, November 16	Hospital dedicates its Dr. R.H. Harte Memorial Nursing School in a new two-story, $56,000 building at Eighth and Delancey Streets.
1940, October 1	Hospital's ambulance service is discontinued and private ambulance providers take its place.
1941	A young intern named C. Everett Koop arrives at the hospital. His service will be interrupted by World War II. Later, he will become surgeon general of the United States.
1941, January 5	Fifty-second Evacuation Hospital (Pennsylvania Hospital Unit) is mobilized for service in World War II. It sees action in the Pacific Theatre.
1942	The busy Emergency Services on the first floor of the Garrett Building is known as "Receive." A former intern describes it as a place where "bleeding and bewildered people trooped into at all hours in a parade of sufficient clinical variety to illustrate medical textbooks of any speciality."
1944, November 1	The first quadruplets born by Caesarean section are delivered. Mrs. Joseph Cirminello, a 118-pound Philadelphia woman, gives birth to three girls and a boy. Doctors knew she was expecting four babies—they had X-rayed her—but they chose not to inform her ahead of time.
1948, Feburary 16	Benjamin Franklin Clinic is opened. It is a group practice, centering on preventative care, a diagnostic clinic that provides periodic and pre-placement medical examinations. It is one of the first such centers on the East Coast.
1948, June	Women's Auxiliary sponsors first Pennsylvania Hospital Day as a fundraiser. The event is held on the hospital grounds at Eighth Street. It will later be held at Independence Hall.
1949	H. Robert Cathcart is hired as assistant administrator. He will spend forty-two years at the hospital, twenty of them as president.
1950	Pennsylvania Hospital becomes more specialized and establishes, in addition to its sophisticated maternity programs, an intensive care unit for neurological patients, a coronary care unit, an orthopedic institute, a diabetes center, a hospice, specialized units in oncology and urology and broadened surgical programs.
1950, April	The Packard Reading Room is named in honor of Dr. Francis R. Packard, who was responsible for creating it in 1940 and for updating the hospital's written history.
1951	Nancy George Boucot, a graduate of the University of Pennsylvania Medical School, is the first female intern at Pennsylvania Hospital.

1951, May 11	Hospital celebrates its 200th anniversary, noting that it has treated more than 2.2 million patients, approximately the population of Philadelphia at that time.
1954, August 16	John A. Hartford Foundation of New York, the legacy of a founder of the Great Atlantic & Pacific Tea Co. (A&P supermarkets) awards the hospital a research grant of $335,000. It is the first of more than a dozen grants that Hartford gives the hospital.
1955, May	Renovations and remodeling are completed at the original Eighth and Pine building.
1957	The relationship between Pennsylvania Hospital and the University of Pennsylvania School of Medicine, which existed informally for nearly two hundred years, is formalized.
1957	The Forty-fourth and Market Street location is closed when Philadelphia exercises the right of eminent domain to bring the subway up through hospital grounds.
1957, July 29	Ground is broken for a $3.3 million, five-story North Building of the Institute at Forty-ninth and Market. All patient facilities are now consolidated into one location known as the Institute of Pennsylvania Hospital.
1959, January 6	North building is opened and dedicated.
1959, January 28–29	Patients are moved from the Forty-fourth Street building to the Forty-ninth Street Building.
1959, February 2–3	Furniture and furnishings are auctioned to the public from the Kirkbride's Forty-fourth Street psychiatric facility.
1959, May 4	Ground is broken for a four-story, $1.1 million nurses' dormitory at Eighth and Spruce.
1960, June 3	Pennsylvania Hospital Day becomes a two-day event with an art show.
1960, September 1	Preston Maternity Hospital is merged with Pennsylvania Hospital. The hospital, originally called Preston Maternity Retreat, dates back to 1866 and was established for "indigent married women of good character."
1962, June 1	First combined men's and women's nursing class graduation.
1964, February 25	The $6 million J. Henry Scheidt Memorial Building at Ninth and Spruce Streets is dedicated.
1965	State's first outpatient community mental health facility is founded at Pennsylvania Hospital—the Hall-Mercer Community Mental Health and Mental Retardation Center. It serves its immediate neighborhood and provides ambulatory services, short-term adult inpatient care, child and family mental health services, developmental disabilities treatment and child development programs. In 1969, the center moves to its own building.

1965, June 22	Hospital is designated a National Historic Landmark by the U.S. Department of Interior, National Park Service.
1965, June 23	Institute of Pennsylvania Hospital is designated a National Historic Landmark by the U.S. Department of Interior, National Park Service.
1965, July	Men's and women's nursing schools are combined.
1966, December 1	Hospital announces plans to build an $8.2 million obstetrics, research and education building.
1967, April 17	The city's first "satellite clinic" is opened by Pennsylvania Hospital. In a movement toward community-based care, the clinic is opened in the Southwark Plaza at Fourth and Washington Streets, and it offers both general medical care and specialized care.
1967, September 18	Construction begins on Hall-Mercer Building at Eighth and Locust Streets.
1967, October	First payroll checks are printed by computer.
1969, April 19	An oral surgery clinic at Eighth Street is named for the late Dr. James R. Cameron.
1969, July 19	Opening of Southeast Philadelphia Neighborhood Health Center at Ninth and South Streets.
1970, January 7	A nursery technician course is initiated, one of the first in the nation.
1970, January 26	Vice president and administrator H. Robert Cathcart is named president of the hospital.
1970, June 10	Pennsylvania Hospital Day awards created.
1971, September 18	Cornerstone set in place in Preston Building. The building houses maternity services, laboratories and educational facilities. It is named for Dr. Jonas Preston, a nineteenth-century Philadelphia obstetrician and philanthropist. In the closing decades of the twentieth century, Pennsylvania Hospital is a source of hope for childless couples, of reassurance to women experiencing high risk pregnancies and of life itself to newborn infants at risk. The hospital's work in reproductive fertility is among the most important being conducted anywhere.
1971, November 16	Relocation of patients from Wards I and II of Pine Building to Spruce Building leaves the Pine Building without any patients for the first time since it was built in 1755.
1971, December 14	First triplets are born in Preston Building.
1972, January 9	Hospital announces that it will phase out its nursing school.
1973, March	Hospital weighs a merger with Jefferson University, ultimately deciding against it because such a partnership might interfere with existing Pennsylvania Hospital programs and would certainly jeopardize the hospital's affiliation with the University of Pennsylvania's School of Medicine.

1976 The hospital's 225th anniversary is celebrated along with the nation's bicentennial. The historical Pine Building is also restored. In preparation for the new Core Building and Gallery Pavillion, and to complete a twenty-five-year development program, the outpatient building is demolished, as well as the Elm Building and its connecting passageways. Design elements from the old structures become a part of the new construction. During this period, the hospital's statue of William Penn is also revitalized at the Center for Archaeometry at Washington University in St. Louis.

1976 At a meeting of the American Hospital Association, H. Robert Cathcart declares that national health insurance is "inevitable." There are not enough funds to provide all the health services needed by the public, Cathcart says.

1976 Friends of the Pennsylvania Hospital help the organization realize a dream long deferred; the Physic Garden is planted. The walled retreat contains about one hundred medicinal plants and is a re-creation of what such a garden would have contained in the eighteenth century. The garden was first authorized in 1774, and was probably deferred for financial reasons.

1976 The Pennsylvania Hospital Insurance Company is organized to provide medical malpractice coverage for its members. The move comes in response to the largest insurer of hospitals in the state fleeing.

1977 A hotline, 215-TEL-MED, is launched to give patients basic health information by phone. Brochures list subjects and operators play tapes at callers' requests on subjects ranging from the emotional experience of the dying to "Little League elbow." Made possible by a $93,000 grant from the William Penn foundation, the tapes are designed to encourage healthcare consumers to take better care of their bodies.

1978 Pennsylvania Hospital is home to the first Antenatal Testing Unit (ATU) in the region.

1979 A grant from the United Way is used to establish a hospice program at Pennsylvania Hospital.

1979 The book *Nurse*, by Peggy Anderson, is published. The *New York Times* bestseller is based on a head nurse at Pennsylvania Hospital, which Anderson researched with the administration's blessing. Later, she would serve on the hospital board.

1980 After a year-long battle, the Dr. Garfield G. Duncan Building, a medical office building behind the hospital, is opened. From the outside, the building appears to be a series of edifices erected between 1835 and 1838, but behind the original fronts, a new structure exists. The hospital had obtained permission to raze the old homes, but protests from neighborhoods caused officials to compromise.

1981 From May through September, an excavation crew digs on the grounds at Eighth and Spruce, unearthing five hundred bags of artifacts, from bedpans and scalpels to bones, test tubes and toothbrushes.

October 8, 1981 The hospital cuts down an elm tree grown from a cutting of the elm under which William Penn signed his famous treaty with the American Indians. Despite efforts to save the tree, which had stood since 1841, it is felled to make way for new construction.

1983, October The new Core Building, later renamed the Cathcart Building, is opened. It is a diamond-shaped, eleven-level structure at the heart of the Eighth and Spruce campus.

1983 First in vitro fertilization pregnancy is achieved.

1985 The first GIFT (gamete intrafallopian transfer) pregnancy in Philadelphia is achieved, laying the groundwork for Pennsylvania Hospital's role in assisted reproductive technologies in the years to come. This is one of the first GIFT programs introduced in the United States.

1986 Pennsylvania Hospital announces a partnership with the Thomas Jefferson University Hospital. The two departments link their orthopedic departments, with Pennsylvania Hospital taking on all joint replacement cases and Jefferson handling all spinal cord and orthopedic trauma cases. Later, a similar arrangement will be devised for otolaryngology.

1986 The Adult Day Health Center is opened. Providing medically supervised daytime care and comprehensive health and rehabilitation services for disabled and chronically ill older adults, it is the first hospital-based adult day care in Philadelphia. The center becomes a leader in the field of adult day care.

1987 Pennsylvania Hospital is home to two obstetrical firsts: the first Birthing Suite in a tertiary care hospital in the state is opened, and the first gestational carrier and egg donor programs in the region are begun to complement Pennsylvania Hospital's existing fertility services.

1992 A milestone in the volume of joint replacements is reached: ten thousand. Pennsylvania Hospital is number one in the country in total joint replacements.

1993 Pennsylvania Hospital announces a new partnership with Thomas Jefferson University Hospital, agreeing to develop formal relationships in the areas of graduate and undergraduate medical education and faculty development. They also promise to enhance cooperation in clinical programs.

1995 Pennsylvania Hospital is the first in the region to achieve one thousand live births from in vitro fertilization, GIFT and other assisted reproductive technologies.

1996 The first Perinatal Evaluation and Treatment Unit (PETU) in the area is staffed by perinatologists to assist in the evaluation of high-risk situations that develop during labor and delivery.

1997 Facing shrinking revenues from insurance providers, the hospital decides to sell its West Philadelphia psychiatric care facility. Behavioral health services, for the first time in over 150 years, are again based at the Eighth Street campus.

1997 Pennsylvania Hospital merges with another historic Philadelphia institution, the University of Pennsylvania Health System, whose roots date back to 1740, when Benjamin Franklin founded the University of Pennsylvania. The move comes in response to sweeping changes in the healthcare arena.

1998 Pennsylvania Hospital becomes home to the Penn Neurological Institute (PNI). The PNI houses the Parkinson's Disease and Movement Disorders Center, which is ranked by *U.S. News and World Report* as the highest in the Philadelphia region and in the top ten nationally for medical and surgical treatments of neurological disorders.

1998 The Women's Imaging Center, which offers mammography, breast ultrasound, stereotactic breast biopsy (a minimally invasive method of monitoring breast lumps) and bone density testing for osteoporosis, is opened. Radiologists interpret results during a woman's initial visit, setting Pennsylvania Hospital apart from its peers in the region.

1998 Nearly 17,600 surgical procedures are performed, ranking Pennsylvania Hospital among the top five most active surgical facilities in the region.

1998 The Center for Bloodless Medicine and Surgery at Pennsylvania Hospital is one of only a few services of its kind on the East Coast, and is the premier provider in the Delaware Valley.

1998 Pennsylvania Hospital is chosen by the City of Philadelphia as one of five places in the region to provide twenty-four-hour emergency psychiatric care. The hospital creates the Crisis Response Center within its Hall-Mercer Community Mental Health Retardation Center.

1999 The Penn Neurological Institute expands with the addition of the ALS Association Center at Pennsylvania Hospital and offers the most comprehensive, current care for ALS (amyotrophic lateral sclerosis, often referred to as Lou Gehrig's disease) patients in the region.

1999	The Joan Karnell Cancer Center at Pennsylvania Hospital moves to its new home, the historic Farm Journal building on Washington Square. The center contains a comprehensive outpatient hematology/oncology service, a state-of-the-art chemotherapy suite and a family education center in a single location.
1999	Pennsylvania Hospital continues to be a regional leader in orthopedic care. Services are provided by Penn Orthopedic Institute, the University of Pennsylvania Health System's faculty practice and Booth Bartolozzi Balderston Orthopedics. Together, they provide services under the brand name of Penn Orthopedics. Penn Orthopedics includes more full-time orthopedic specialists than any program in the region, and these doctors perform more orthopedic procedures, including total knee replacements, than anyone else in the area.
2000	The Joint Commission for Accreditation of Healthcare Organizations sends the following message to the hospital on the completion of its year 2000 survey: "The team would like to express to your staff our finding of their exceptional dedication to their hospital and patients. You have created a model of quality and caring for both your patients and the community you serve."
2000	Pennsylvania Hospital considerably expands its rehabilitation services by creating an acute inpatient unit in the hospital and an outpatient rehabilitation center for patients with movement disorders in the Penn Neurological Institute.
2001, February	The University of Pennsylvania announces plans to spin off its health system, including Pennsylvania Hospital, into a separate, affiliated nonprofit organization instead of selling the financially troubled network.
2001, May 11	Pennsylvania Hospital celebrates its 250th anniversary. The hospital plans parties, tours and health fairs.
2003	*U.S. News and World Report* ranks Pennsylvania Hospital as one of the top ten hospitals in America.
2004	The hospital adds technology that allows patients who speak languages other than English to communicate with hospital personnel over the phone. Many Spanish, Vietnamese, Russian, Mandarin and Cambodian speakers use the service.
2004	A study in AARP *Modern Maturity* ranks Pennsylvania Hospital as one of the top ten hospitals in America. The hospital receives additional honors for cardiac care, cardio-vascular surgeries, infectious care, knee-hip orthopedics and pulmonary care—all five specialties are also ranked within the top ten in the nation.

2006 Benjamin Franklin's 300th birthday is celebrated in grand style at the hospital he helped found.

2006 Kathleen Kinslow, CRNA, EdD, MBA, is named executive director of the hospital. She is the first female executive director in the hospital's history.

2006 Hospital officials announce their intention to raise $2 million to fund critical repairs on the Pine Building and $5 million to begin an endowment to pay for regular preservation and maintenance.

2006 The "Learn to Grow" program is launched. The program uses the Physic Garden to teach area schoolchildren about the history of herbal medicine and its contributions to science and society.

2006 Dr. Robert E. Booth, chief of orthopedic surgery at Pennsylvania Hospital, introduces the Gender Solutions High-Flex Knee, based on three distinct shape differences between men's and women's knees. The implant is designed to alleviate knee pain and restore mobility, while offering fit and function tailored for female patients.

2007 The hospital is awarded a $350,000 grant to help fund the restoration of the Pine Building. The money comes from the National Park Service/National Trust for Historic Preservation's Save America's Treasures program.

2007 The hospital continues to amass honors. *U.S. News and World Report* ranks Pennsylvania Hospital among the best in the nation for orthopedic care. *Philadelphia Magazine* recognizes twenty-seven Pennsylvania Hospital physicians as "Top Docs."

2007 Between 1765 and 2007, 268,286 people are born at Pennsylvania Hospital; 5,107 births were recorded in 2007 alone.

NOTES

THE EARLY HOSPITAL, 1751–1800

1. Francis R. Packard and Florence M. Greim, *Some Account of The Pennsylvania Hospital of Philadelphia, from 1751 to 1938. With a Continuation of the Account to Year 1956* (Philadelphia: The Pennsylvania Hospital, 1957), v.
2. Ibid.
3. Todd Savage, "Oldest Living Hospital Tells All," *Hospitals and Health Networks*, July 5, 1998, 49–52.
4. William H. Williams, "The Early Days of Anglo-America's First Hospital," *Journal of the American Medical Association* 220, 1 (April 3, 1972).
5. *Pennsylvania Gazette*, March 18, 1731.
6. Ibid., August 8, 1751.
7. John E. Ransom, "The Beginnings of Hospitals in the United States," *Bulletin of the History of Medicine* 13 (1943).
8. William H. Williams, "The 'Industrious Poor' and the Founding of Pennsylvania Hospital," *The Pennsylvania Magazine of History and Biography* 97, 4 (October 1973): 431–43.
9. William H. Williams, "The Pennsylvania Hospital, 1751–1801: An Internal Examination of Anglo-America's First Hospital" (PhD diss., University of Delaware, 1972), 60–64.
10. Ibid., 66–68.
11. Kenneth R. Crain, "Some Account of the Pennsylvania Hospital, from its first rise to the beginning of the year 1951," *Hospital Management* (January 1951): 5.
12. Sydney P. Clark, *Pennsylvania Hospital—Since May 11, 1751: Two Hundred Years in Philadelphia* (New York: The Newcomen Society in North America, 1951), 5–10.
13. Thomas G. Morton, *The History of the Pennsylvania Hospital, 1751–1895* (Philadelphia: Philadelphia Times Printing House, 1897), 440–43.
14. "Pennsylvania Hospital's History In Brief," internal Pennsylvania Hospital Memo, 1961.
15. Morton, *History*, 208–11.
16. Packard and Greim, *Some Account*, 1–12.
17. Morton, *History*, 211.
18. Ibid., 525.
19. Benjamin Franklin, *Some Account of the Pennsylvania Hospital; From Its First Rise to the Beginning of the Fifth Month, Called May, 1754* (Philadelphia: printed at the office of the United States' gazette, 1817), 53–55.

20. Morton, *History*, 525–31.
21. Packard and Greim, *Some Account*, 17–21.
22. Edmond G. Thomas, "Pennsylvania Hospital's 200 Years," *Hospitals: Journal of the American Hospital Association* (May 1951).
23. William H. Williams, *America's First Hospital: The Pennsylvania Hospital, 1751–1841* (Wayne, PA: Haverford House Publishers, 1976), 31–33.
24. Morton, *History*, 222–24.
25. Packard and Greim, *Some Account*, 31.
26. Williams, *America's First Hospital*, 44–47.
27. Ibid.
28. Crain, "Some Account," 3–22.
29. Dorothy I. Lansing, "Jacob Ehrenzeller, 1757–1838," section on medical history, College of Physicians, 1976.
30. Williams, *America's First Hospital*, 57–61.
31. Ibid., 65–66.
32. Crain, "Some Account," 3–22.
33. Morton, *History*, 203–06.
34. Williams, *America's First Hospital*, 70.
35. Packard and Greim, *Some Account*, 32.
36. Williams, *America's First Hospital*, 68–83.
37. Ibid., 73.
38. Ibid., 68–83.
39. Packard and Greim, *Some Account*, 71–75.
40. Williams, *America's First Hospital*, 84–103.
41. Crain, "Some Account," 3–22.
42. Ibid.
43. Williams, *America's First Hospital*, 104–07.
44. Morton, *History*, 127–28.
45. Williams, *America's First Hospital*, 64–65.
46. Ibid.
47. Ibid., 115.
48. Ibid., 146–47.
49. Ibid., 81–82.
50. Morton, *History*, 164–65.
51. Steven M. Spencer, "They Didn't Know What They Started," *Saturday Evening Post*, February 24, 1951.
52. Morton, *History*, 494.
53. Ibid., 134.
54. Howard Sudak, "Pennsylvania Hospital's Legacy on the Field of Psychiatry," www.uphs.upenn.edu/paharc/features/paharc.html.
55. "A Brief History of The Institute of Pennsylvania Hospital," Pennsylvania Hospital memo, December 9, 1976.
56. "Institute Archives Recall Kirkbride's Hospital," *Pennsylvania Hospital Quill* (May/June 1975): 1–2.
57. *Philadelphia Inquirer*, April 16, 1991.
58. Jack D. Pressman, "Making Psychiatry Respectable: Earl Bond, Edward Strecker, Kenneth Appel, and the Institute of Pennsylvania Hospital," *Transactions and Studies of the College of Physicians of Philadelphia* 13, 4 (1991): 425–43.

59. "A Brief History of The Institute of Pennsylvania Hospital."
60. Pressman, "Making Psychiatry Respectable," 435–440.
61. *Philadelphia Inquirer*, April 16, 1991.
62. "Dr. Thomas Story Kirkbride," http://www.uphs.upenn.edu/paharc/timeline/1801/tline14.html.
63. "Joseph Hughes M.D.: He helped create history at The Institute," *Pennsylvania Hospital Quill* (Spring 1979).
64. "Mental Health Facility," http://www.uphs.upenn.edu/paharc/timeline/1951/tline20.html.
65. "Teenagers at Institute Face Reality Daily…At School," *Pennsylvania Hospital Quill* (March/April 1972).
66. "Special Education: The Mill Creek School," http://pennhealth.com/behav_health/services/pahosp/special.html.
67. *Philadelphia Inquirer*, October 3, 1996.
68. "History of Pennsylvania Hospital: Historic Library," www.uphs.upenn.edu/paharc/timeline/1751/tline4.html.
69. Morton, *History*, 345–64.
70. "History of Pennsylvania Hospital: Historic Library."
71. Williams, *America's First Hospital*, 86–87.

THE GROWING HOSPITAL, 1800–1951

72. Charles E. Rosenberg, *The Care of Strangers: The Rise of America's First Hospital System* (New York: Basic Books, Inc. 1978), 4–18.
73. Williams, *America's First Hospital*, 130–32.
74. "Pennsylvania Hospital's History In Brief," internal Pennsylvania Hospital Memo, 1961.
75. Williams, *America's First Hospital*, 145–46.
76. Alfred Henderson, "A Note on the 'Circular Room' of the Pennsylvania Hospital," *Journal of the History of Medicine* 19 (April 1964): 156–60.
77. Ibid.
78. Morton, *History*, 497.
79. Clark, *Pennsylvania Hospital*, 24–25.
80. Ibid.
81. Morton, *History*, 63.
82. Williams, *America's First Hospital*, 133–34.
83. M. Adelaide Nutting and Lavinia L. Dock, *A History of Nursing* (New York: G.P. Putnam's Sons, 1920), 336–38.
84. "Women's Auxiliary Begins New Chapter in its Long History," *Pennsylvania Hospital Quill* (November/December 1970).
85. Rosenberg, *Care of Strangers*, 22.
86. Ibid., 24.
87. Ibid.
88. Williams, *America's First Hospital*, 124–47.

89. "Civil War, 1861–1865," http://www.uphs.upenn.edu/paharc/timeline/1851/tline15.html.
90. Packard and Greim, *Some Account*, 31–34.
91. "Civil War, 1861–1865."
92. Packard and Greim, *Some Account*, 44–45.
93. Joel D. Howell, "Machines and Medicine: Technology Transforms the American Hospital," in *The American General Hospital: Communities and Social Contexts*, edited by Diana Elizabeth and Janet Golden (Ithaca, NY: Cornell University Press, 1989.)
94. "Spanish-American War," http://www.uphs.upenn.edu/paharc/timeline/1851/tline17.html.
95. Lester S. King, "Clinical Laboratories Become Important, 1870–1900," *Journal of the American Medical Association* 249, 22 (June 10, 1983): 3025–29.
96. Richard H. Harte, *Pennsylvania Hospital Unit In the Great War* (New York: Paul B. Hoeber, 1921), 11–31.
97. Packard and Greim, *Some Account*, 128–30.
98. "World War I, 1917–1918," http://www.uphs.upenn.edu/paharc/timeline/1901/tline18.html.
99. Isaac Starr, "Influenza in 1918: Reflections of the Epidemic in Philadelphia," *Annals of Internal Medicine* 85 (1976): 516–18.
100. Morton, *History*, 107.
101. Packard and Greim, *Some Account*, 110–11.
102. Joseph Vander Veer, *History of Pennsylvania Hospital Unit in World War II (Evacuation Station #52, Station Hospital #364)* (Bryn Mawr, PA: Dorrance and Co., 1989), 1–6.
103. Ibid., 7–188.
104. Ann Pekarik Stasheff, interview, March 24, 2008.
105. 193rd Annual Report of Pennsylvania Hospital.
106. "Benjamin Franklin Clinic: An Unlikely Infant Begins Its 30th Year," Benjamin Franklin Clinic news release, spring 1977.
107. Clark, *Pennsylvania Hospital*, 34–35.
108. Dr. Robert Gill, interview, March 25, 2008.
109. Peter A. Gearhart, "Notes on the History of Obstetrics and Gynecology at Pennsylvania Hospital" (paper presented at the S. Leon Israel, MD Memorial Symposium, June 13, 2002).
110. Ibid.
111. Dr. Richard Norris and Dr. John C. Hirst, "The Preston Retreat," handout article, 1936.
112. Gearhart, "Notes."
113. Marsha F. Goldsmith, "At Pennsylvania Hospital, 250 Years of Care," *Journal of the American Medical Association* 285, 18 (May 9, 2001): 2313–16.
114. Penn OB/GYN care, "http://pennhealth.com/obgyn/services/obstetrics/midwifery.html."
115. Anne L. Austin, *History of Nursing Source Book* (New York: G.P. Putnam's Sons, 1957), 347.
116. Williams, *America's First Hospital*, 6–7.
117. Crain, "Some Account," 3–22.
118. Williams, *America's First Hospital*, 112.
119. Ibid., 55–56.
120. Ibid., 111–13.

121. Nutting and Dock, *History of Nursing*, 338.
122. Morton, *History*, 104–07.
123. "Annual Lucy Walker Lecture," press release, Pennsylvania Hospital, September 25, 1968.
124. Patricia O'Brien, "'All a Woman's Life Can Bring': the Domestic Roots of Nursing in Philadephia, 1830–1885," *Nursing Research* 36, 1 (January/February 1987): 12–16.
125. "School of Nursing, 1875–1974," www.uphs.upenn.edu/paharc/timeline/1851/tline16.html.
126. Ann Pekarik Stasheff, interview, March 24, 2008.
127. "School of Nursing to Close in 1974," *Pennsylvania Hospital Quill* (July/August 1972): 1.
128. Peggy Anderson, "'Person After Person Steered Me to Pennsy,'" *Pennsylvania Hospital Quill* (Winter 1979).
129. Packard and Greim, *Some Account*, 87–89.
130. Ibid., 87–89.
131. "A Virtual Tour," http://www.uphs.upenn.edu/paharc/tour/tour3.html.
132. Packard and Greim, *Some Account*, 90–91.
133. "The Rittenhouse Clock: An Old Friend Returns to Pennsylvania Hospital," *Pennsylvania Hospital Quill* (March/April 1975).
134. Packard and Greim, *Some Account*, 92–96.
135. "The Physic Garden of Pennsylvania Hospital," internal pamphlet, undated.
136. "Hospital to get a Botanical Garden—200 Years Later," *Pennsylvania Hospital Quill* (March/April 1975).

THE CONTEMPORARY HOSPITAL, 1951–PRESENT

137. William B. Kennedy, letter to of the Intern Department, Pennsylvania Hospital, December 19, 1950.
138. John N. Hatfield, letter to William B. Seymour, director of administration, University Hospitals of Cleveland, October 29, 1951.
139. H. Robert Cathcart, interview, September 28, 2007.
140. Dr. Robert Gill, interview, November 2, 2007.
141. Ibid.
142. Ibid.
143. Dr. Terrence Malloy, interview, December 14, 2007.
144. Ibid.
145. H. Robert Cathcart, interview.
146. Ibid.
147. *Philadelphia Inquirer*, September 9, 1991.
148. Dr. Robert Gill, interview, November 2, 2007.
149. Morris Cheston Jr., interview, September 26, 2007.
150. *Philadelphia Inquirer*, September 9, 1991.
151. *Philadelphia Bulletin*, March 29, 1973.
152. H. Robert Cathcart, interview, September 28, 2007.

153. "How DRGs Work at Pennsylvania Hospital," *Pennsylvania Hospital Quill* (Summer/Fall 1984).
154. *Philadelphia Inquirer*, October 27, 1996.
155. Ibid., October 3, 1996.
156. *Philadelphia Daily News*, January 14, 1997.
157. *Philadelphia Business Journal*, May 17, 2002.
158. *Philadelphia Inquirer*, February 18, 1997.
159. *Philadelphia Business Journal*, August 6, 2004.
160. Ibid., March 22, 1996.
161. *Philadelphia Inquirer*, October 27, 1996.
162. Ibid., November 13, 1996.
163. Dr. Michael Buckley, interview, September 28, 2007.
164. Pennsylvania Hospital 246th Annual Report to the Community for the Year 1997.
165. *Philadelphia Inquirer*, November 13, 1996.
166. *Philadelphia Business Journal*, March 3, 1997.
167. Ibid., May 9, 1997.
168. Ibid., April 13, 2001.
169. *Daily Pennsylvanian*, October 5, 1999.
170. *Philadelphia Inquirer*, November 2, 1999.
171. *Philadelphia Daily News*, October 22, 1999.
172. *Philadelphia Inquirer*, July 20, 1999.
173. Morris Cheston Jr., interview, September 26, 2007.
174. *Philadelphia Inquirer*, November 2, 1999.
175. Kathleen Kinslow, interview, September 18, 2007.
176. Morris Cheston Jr., interview, September 26, 2007.
177. Ibid.
178. Ibid.
179. Dr. Terrence Malloy, interview, December 14, 2007.
180. *Philadelphia Business Journal*, May 4, 2007.
181. Morris Cheston Jr., interview, September 26, 2007.
182. Dr. Michael Buckley, interview, September 28, 2007.
183. Kathleen Kinslow, interview, September 18, 2007.
184. Dr. Michael Buckley, interview, September 28, 2007.
185. Ibid.
186. Ibid.
187. Dr. Terrence Malloy, interview, December 14, 2007.